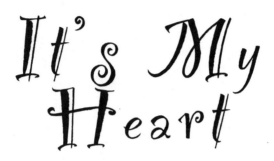

It's My Heart

The World's Leading Guide to Congenital Heart Defects for Patients and Parents

Revised Edition

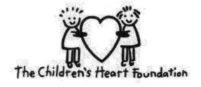

The Children's Heart Foundation

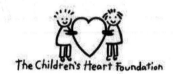

The Children's Heart Foundation

www.childrensheartfoundation.org

(888) 248-8140

ISBN: 0-9841447-9-2

$\mathcal{T}able\ of\ \mathcal{C}ontents$

Introduction

It's My Heart

This free resource is for patients and families affected by congenital and acquired heart disease. It is a guide to be used with medical professionals. It is not a substitute for your child's physician. Never hesitate to direct any questions or concerns about your child's heart problem to your pediatric cardiologist…no question is too simple or silly. You know your child better than anyone. Don't be shy about calling your child's physician to discuss any concerns. If your child looks different, acts different, or is having difficulty eating, always call.

Also, know that you are not alone. Approximately 40,000 babies are born in the United States each year with congenital heart defects. That represents about one in every 125 births, topping the list as America's most prevalent birth defect. There are many ways in which the heart can develop abnormalities. Genetic and environmental factors have been linked to congenital heart disease. But in most cases, the cause is unknown. The good news is that most people who have childhood heart surgery grow up to be healthy adults. But it is important to get the heart care that you need to keep well. If your heart defect is listed as complex, experts recommend that you get life-long care from experts in congenital heart disease. This is true even if you had successful surgery in childhood.

It's My Heart is intended to provide you with information on some of the many issues you may be dealing with since your child was diagnosed with a congenital heart defect. The book was written by doctors, nurses and parents in a collaborative effort spearheaded by The Children's Heart Foundation (CHF) in Lincolnshire, Illinois. Neither the book nor the Foundation are directly associated with any one hospital or institution.

The National Board of Directors of The Children's Heart Foundation wishes to thank the following individuals for their commitment and generosity in providing information, time and resources to the development of *It's My Heart:*

It's My Heart Project Committee: Thomas Weigel, M.D.; Carl Backer, M.D.; Marla Mendelson, M.D.; Hilton Hudson, M.D.; Julie Creaden, CPNP; Betsy Peterson, CHF Founder; Jena Rausch, publisher; Barbra Armaroli, first-edition editor; and CHF staff members Rosemary Wheeler, Christina Larson and Ellen Weiss.

Chapter Authors and Illustrators: Alexander J. Muster, M.D.; Katherine A. Tubeszewski, RN, MSN; Lynn C. Graham, RN, BSN; Katherine Kerrigan, RN, MS, CPNP; Maggie Fischer, RN, MS; Jennifer Cleary, RN, MS; Linda Hellstedt, MSN, RN; Sue Rushmore; Natalie Rudolph, RN, MSN; Betsy Peterson; illustrations are used by permission of John Wiley & Sons, Inc.; *Congenital Heart Disease: A Diagrammatic Atlas* by Charles E. Mullins, M.D. and David C. Mayer, M.D., Copyright © 1988 WileyLiss, Inc.; Medtronic, Inc.

The Children's Heart Foundation also wishes to thank the Northwestern University Dance Marathon 2011 for its generous support of the second edition of the book, as well as Medtronic Foundation for its support for funding the initial production and distribution of this book; the Gerber Foundation, WNUA Cares for Kids Foundation, Circle of Service Foundation, Inc., and the Winnetka Rotary for funding the development of the book; Amanda Haley for the beautiful and unique *It's My Heart* logo; Andrea Wilhelm, AHW Design, for layout and design; Angela Vennemann for updated layout; and Hilton Hudson, M.D., and the team at Hilton Publishing, Inc.

The Children's Heart Foundation was founded in 1996. Its mission is to raise funds to support research toward discovering the causes of and improving the methods of diagnosing, treating and preventing congenital heart defects. The Children's Heart Foundation is a 501(c)(3) tax-exempt charitable organization. CHF is not affiliated with any one medical institution or organization. This allows funds to be directed to the most promising research anywhere in the world, under the direction of our Medical Advisory Board.

About this Book

When the first edition of **It's My Heart** was published in 2004, it addressed a dire need noted by patients with congenital heart defects and their parents and families. Although doctors and nurses often explained things well, written materials were either too simple (pamphlets on how the normal heart works) or too complex (medical journals). What was needed was a book with clear writing and illustrations on the most common kinds of heart defects, tests, equipment, surgical procedures and medications.

It's My Heart was the answer to that need, and it became an immediate success! Notable is CHF's decision from the start to make the book available free for families and to post the entire contents of the book on its website for free reading or downloading. Countless people around the world have benefited from the book in its English and Spanish versions.

For this revised edition of **It's My Heart,** the entire contents have been reviewed and, where needed, updated with the latest in medical information.

Contact CHF at www.childrensheartfoundation.org or (888) 248-8140 for further information on the organization's activities throughout the United States.

To view a current roster of CHF's Medical Advisory Board, visit www.childrensheartfoundation.org/about-chf/officers-boards-staff.

The Normal Heart

The heart has two roles. First, it delivers oxygen-rich blood to all living tissues in the body. Second, it recirculates used blood (in which the oxygen has been replaced by carbon dioxide) through the lungs, where carbon dioxide is exhaled and replaced by oxygen that has been inhaled.

Arteries carry blood away from the heart and veins return blood to the heart.

Development of the Normal Heart and Vessels

During the first seven weeks after conception, known as the *embryonic period*, the heart completes development from a single straight tube into a complicated four-chambered pump containing four valves. From then until the baby is born, the *fetal period*, the heart and the vessels grow in size. Until a newborn takes its first breath after clamping of the umbilical cord, the lungs are not functional. The mother's placenta serves as the lung while the baby is in the womb. The oxygen-rich (pink) blood from the placenta refreshes the oxygen-poor (blue) blood in the fetus and this mixed blood is then propelled through the heart to the fetus's body tissues. Although this mixed blood is low in oxygen, it is tolerated well by the fetus. After delivery, the lungs begin to function; the communication passages, or shunts, that allowed mixing of the blue and pink blood while the baby was still in the womb, spontaneously close over time. The two blood streams—the blue and the pink—are then separated and the newborn turns pink.

Thus, circulation in the normal newborn consists of two completely separated paths: the right (blue or venous) side and the left (pink or arterial) side. The left side propels the fresh arterial blood to every living cell in the body in order to supply oxygen and nutrients, and to pick up carbon dioxide and waste products. The used venous blood turns dark (oxygen depleted, blue, cyanotic) and is recirculated by the right side through the lungs. The blue blood passes through tiny blood vessels in the lung called capillaries, where oxygen is drawn from air sacs and carbon dioxide is removed from the blood. The refreshed pink blood is picked up by the left side and propelled into all body tissues to sustain life.

Structure and Function of the
Normal Heart and Vessels

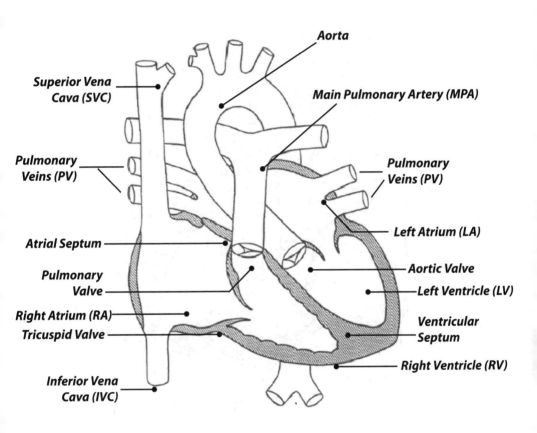

*Use this illustration of the normal heart to ask your child's physician
about your child's defect and the necessary correction*

Anatomy and Function of the Normal Heart

The normal heart (see figure) is composed of two muscular blood pumps, the right and left ventricles, joined by a common wall. The blood enters and exits the two pumps without crossing the wall and each pump supplies a separate system: (a) the lung, or pulmonary, circulation, and (b) the body, or systemic, circulation. The non-pumping components of the heart contribute to its efficiency as a forward pump.

Pulmonary Circulation

The right side of the heart is responsible for lung, or pulmonary, circulation. It consists of two large collecting veins, the superior and inferior vena cava (SVC and IVC), that return the oxygen-depleted blood to the right upper collecting chamber of the heart, the right atrium (RA). The blood then enters the right pumping chamber, the right ventricle (RV), and is propelled into the common lung artery, the main pulmonary artery (MPA), that divides into the right and left pulmonary artery branch. The branching continues within the lungs until tiny capillary vessels wrap around the air sacs where oxygen is exchanged for carbon dioxide.

Systemic Circulation

The left side of the heart is responsible for body, or systemic, circulation. The process begins with two right and two left pulmonary veins (PV) that collect the fresh blood from the lungs and fill the left upper collecting chamber of the heart, the left atrium (LA). The blood then enters the left pumping chamber of the heart, the left ventricle (LV), and is propelled into the largest body artery, the aorta (AO). The aorta branches into many smaller arteries that continue branching until, as tiny capillary vessels, they reach all body tissues, where they distribute oxygen and nutrients and pick up waste products. After this point, the oxygen-depleted capillaries turn blue, become veins and deliver the used blood to the right side of the heart. The process is repeated with each heart beat.

Valves

Four valves in the heart assure that the blood flows in the correct direction. The right inlet valve, called the *tricuspid valve*, between the right atrium and the right ventricle, opens to fill the ventricle and then closes to prevent the blood from flowing backward, often referred to as regurgitation. The right exit valve, the *pulmonic valve,* between the right ventricle and the main pulmonary artery, opens to fill the pulmonary artery, in which the blood flows to the lung, and then closes to prevent regurgitation of the blood back into the right ventricle. The left inlet valve, the *mitral valve,* between the left atrium and the left ventricle, opens to fill the left ventricle and then closes to prevent backflow of the blood. The left exit valve, the aortic valve, between the left ventricle and the aorta, opens to fill the aorta and then closes to prevent regurgitation of the blood back into the left ventricle.

Aorta

The aorta is composed of three parts: the ascending aorta, which directs blood up toward the head; the aortic arch, which curves from upward to downward; and the descending aorta, which directs blood down toward the lower body. Two coronary arteries arise from the ascending aorta, at the aortic root close to the heart, and supply the heart muscle with fresh blood.

Pulse

Each heartbeat, or pulse, consists of two separate ventricular activities: 1) systole (pronounced SIS-toe-lee) the contraction or squeezing that forces the exit valve to open, the inlet valve to close, and the blood to fill the artery; and 2) diastole (pronounced die-ASS-toe-lee) the relaxation of the heart that occurs when the inlet valve opens to permit the ventricle to refill and the exit valve closes. The arterial pulse, usually felt at the wrist, is related to systole. The arterial blood pressure, usually measured in the upper arm, has a systolic value, the higher number, and a diastolic value, the lower number.

Natural Pacemaker

Each heartbeat is triggered by a faint electrical current generated by a natural pacemaker, a lifetime battery-like tissue, called the sinus node, at the top of the right upper chamber. A normal sinus node generates a slow heart rate at rest that can speed up when needed and is regular in rhythm, a normal sinus rhythm. The electrical current spreads from the right atrium to an area on the wall between the ventricles, called the atrio-ventricular node, where it passes through microscopic wiring, beginning as a common bundle and dividing into two-bundle branches, to the ventricles where it activates the muscles to con tract, in systole. The sinus node and the atrio-ventricular node are controlled by the involuntary nervous system of the brain(autonomic nervous system) through nerve connections from the brain to the nodes directly. Thus, the brain controls the patient's heart rate.

Blood Pressure

The heart contracts to generate just enough tension, or systolic pressure, within the ventricles to maintain normal forward flow. The right exit valve, the pulmonary valve, related to lung circulation, requires low pressure to open. Thus, the right ventricle pressure is normally low. The left exit valve, the aortic valve, related to systemic circulation, requires about four times as much pressure as the right valve requires to open, hence the normal left ventricular systolic pressure is relatively high. During ventricular refilling or diastole, when the chamber relaxes, the pressure drops to the low level that is present in the veins and upper chambers. This is the diastolic pressure. In the pulmonary artery and in the aorta, the systolic pressure is normally identical to that in the respective ventricles, whereas the arterial diastolic pressure is higher than the ventricular diastolic pressure to keep the exit valve closed while the ventricle is refilling.

Protective Layers

The heart is wrapped and separated from the surrounding organs by a double-layered, thin, smooth, and lubricated membrane called the pericardium. The inside of the heart chambers is lined with a thin membrane-like layer of cells called the endocardium. The muscular part of each ventricle is called the myocardium.

Types of Abnormal Heart Disease

There are two categories of heart abnormalities—congenital and acquired. Congenital heart disease (CHD) means the child is born with an abnormally structured heart and/or large vessels. Such hearts may have incomplete or missing parts, may be put together the wrong way, may have holes between chamber partitions or may have narrow or leaky valves or narrow vessels. (See Chapter Two for more discussion of various forms of CHD.) Some CHDs may have genetic or environmental causes. With acquired heart disease, the child is born with a normal heart that malfunctions at a later time in life. Such hearts may pump poorly, be too stiff, infected, or may beat too fast, too slowly or too erratically. While most acquired heart disease occurs in adults, such as coronary and hypertensive heart disease, some children acquire heart disease, usually due to bacterial or viral infections. (*See Chapter Three for more discussion of various forms of acquired heart disease.*)

Congenital Heart Defects

There are many types of congenital heart defects, ranging from those that pose a relatively small threat to the health of the child to those that require immediate surgery. This chapter reviews many types of congenital heart defects and the surgical procedures your physician may recommend to correct the condition.

Aortic Stenosis

Aortic stenosis is a narrowing or obstruction in the aorta, the largest blood vessel in the body, which serves as a passageway for pink oxygen-rich blood to leave the heart and to get pumped out to the body. Any obstruction in the aorta requires that the heart muscle must work harder to get blood out of the heart.

Aortic stenosis can occur in one or more of three areas of the aorta: subvalvar, below the aortic valve; valvar, having to do with the aortic valve itself; or, supravalvar, above the aortic valve. Each type of obstruction requires a different type of repair and can occur congenitally or develop at any time during a person's life.

The most common type of aortic stenosis occurs when the aortic valve is not properly formed. Normally, the aortic valve has three leaflets or flaps. These flaps open each time the heart pumps and close when the heart pauses between pumps to form a tight seal so blood does not leak back into the heart. Sometimes, the valve has only two leaflets (bicuspid) instead of three (tricuspid). Sometimes, the leaflets are fused together so the valve cannot open all the way. And sometimes, the entire valve may be significantly smaller than it should be, known as hypoplastic. In all three types of valve problems, the aortic valve may be leaky, or regurgitant.

Aortic valve stenosis may be severe from the moment a baby is born, if the baby's heart has already been doing extra work before birth. Symptoms of early heart failure may include fast breathing, difficulty with feeding, fast heart rate and low blood pressure.

More commonly, aortic valve stenosis is relatively mild in early life, and the baby may appear to be completely healthy, the only symptom being a mild heart murmur. Many times, the child with mild aortic stenosis does not require immediate treatment. Periodic visits to the cardiologist may provide the information necessary to determine when or if treatment is necessary.

If treatment for aortic valve stenosis is required, the cardiologist may first recommend a catheter balloon aortic valve procedure. **(A)** A deflated balloon is inserted into the large artery in the child's leg at the groin. The balloon is advanced up the artery into the aorta and across the aortic valve. Once the balloon is positioned across the aortic valve, it can be inflated to force open the leaflets of the aortic valve. This procedure, usually done under sedation in the cardiac catheterization lab, may relieve the stenosis temporarily or for many years.

If the aortic valve is very leaky, the cardiologist may recommend a surgical repair. With this procedure, the child will be placed on a heart-lung machine, so the surgeon can work on the aortic valve leaflets to make them as normal as possible.

In all cases of aortic valve stenosis, the child will need to see a cardiologist throughout his or her life to make sure the valve continues to work well. Abnormal heart valves that have been successfully repaired may not continue to work well as the heart grows and develops. It is not uncommon for a valve to require replacement later in life.

Aortic valve replacement is not an appealing choice in children for three important reasons. First, there is no valve replacement that will grow with a child. The younger the child is when the valve is replaced, the more operations will be needed as the child outgrows the valve. In addition, as the child grows new bone, calcium deposits may occur on a replacement valve, causing the leaflets to malfunction. Second, when a mechanical artificial valve is used, the child must receive anticoagulation medication to reduce the blood's natural clotting action. This type of medication requires frequent blood testing to adjust for dosage. Moreover, physical activity will have to be limited, as the medication will cause the child to bleed excessively with any injury. Third, there are no valves small

enough to fit an infant; a child must be several years of age before valve replacement surgery is even considered. As a result, to avoid aortic valve replacement
in children, a pediatric cardiologist may recommend valve balloonings or repairs
to postpone valve replacement surgery as long as possible.

Surgeons may consider one other option besides mechanical valve replacement when the aortic valve continues to work poorly after several attempts
to repair it. This procedure, called the Ross procedure, is open-heart surgery
in which the child's own pulmonary valve is used to replace the abnormal
aortic valve. The pulmonary valve is then replaced with a tissue valve, such as
from a pig or cow or human cadaver. The tissue artificial valve does not cause
blood clots like the mechanical valve and therefore does not require anticoagulation medication. Plus, it usually lasts longer than mechanical replacements
in the pulmonary position and therefore hopefully requires fewer replacement procedures later in life. A great appeal to the Ross procedure surgical
approach is that with the recent advent of pulmonary valve replacement by
catheterization, subsequent procedures on the pulmonary valve can be done
via cardiac catheter as opposed to an open-heart procedure.

In addition to aortic valve stenosis, two other types of aortic narrowing or obstruction can occur. In subaortic stenosis, **(B)** the narrowing or obstruction occurs as
blood leaves the left ventricle and before it reaches the aortic valve. As in aortic
valve stenosis, this defect may appear to be quite mild early in life, with the only
symptom being a heart murmur, although the condition tends to progress with age.

Subaortic stenosis is repaired in one of several ways, all of which require open-
heart surgery. If the obstruction below the aortic valve is caused by membrane,
tissue or extra muscle, the obstruction can be resected or cut to open the area
below the valve. If however, the area below the valve is narrowed in a tunnel-
like fashion, a patch enlargement is required, using a manmade material called
Gore-Tex in a procedure called the modified Konno procedure.

In supravalvar aortic stenosis, **(C)** the narrowing or "waist" occurs in the aorta
above the valve. This relatively uncommon form of aortic stenosis is repaired
surgically using a Gore-Tex patch to enlarge the narrowed area.

(A)

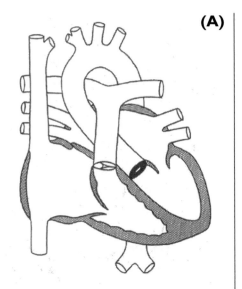

Valvular
Aortic Stenosis

(B)

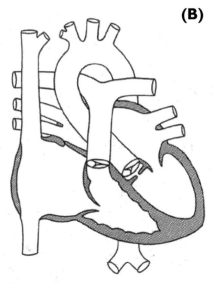

Discrete Membranous
Subaortic Stenosis

(C)

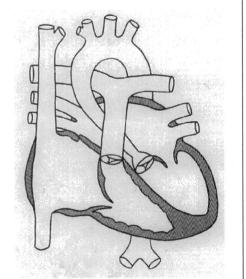

Supravalvular
Aortic Stenosis

Normal Heart

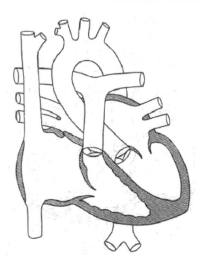

Please refer to page 11 for a detailed
illustration of the normal heart.

Atrial Septal Defect (ASD)

In a normal heart, the right and left heart chambers are completely separated by a solid wall called the septum. An *atrial septal defect* (ASD) is a hole in the septum between the right and left upper collecting chambers of the heart, the atria. This hole allows a stream of pink blood from the left atrium to cross over into the right atrium and to mix with the blue blood. Consequently, an increased amount of blood flows through the right heart chambers and the pulmonary artery leading to the lungs. This added stream of fully oxygenated pink blood recirculating through the lung vessels is a wasted effort as no further oxygen can be picked up. Depending on the location of the hole, these defects have different names:

Ostium Secundum Defects are the most common and are often located in the center of the septum. Occasionally, there are multiple small openings, or the hole can be located somewhat off center.

Ostium Primum Defects are low in the septum and adjacent to the tricuspid and mitral inlet. This can cause the mitral valve to be malformed or cleft, which may cause the valve to be regurgitant. With each beat of the heart, pink blood from the left ventricle leaks back into both the left and right atria causing excessive chamber enlargement and adding more volume to the already overloaded lung circulation system. Ostium primum defects are a type of endocardial cushion defect. When associated with a cleft mitral valve, they are considered a partial atrioventricular canal.

Sinus Venosus Defects lie close to the entry of the great veins, or venae cavae, into the right atrium. Defects that are near the superior vena cava at the top of the atrial septum are often complicated by inappropriate attachment of the right-sided pulmonary veins to the superior vena cava or the right atrium. This condition is called anomalous pulmonary venous connection.

Probe Patent Foramen Ovale (FO) is an incompletely closed flap between the atria. This flap is widely open in the normal fetal heart, but seals itself off in the first few months after birth. When the flap is patent (open), it usually remains undetected and harmless. Rarely, it can be associated with transient stroke or migraines in adult life, due to thrombus embolization to the systemic circulation, in which case, it requires closure.

Symptoms and Treatment

Atrial septal defect (ASD) symptoms depend on the size of the hole, the number of holes and the extent of associated abnormalities. Smaller defects may cause few if any symptoms during childhood. Large defects may cause exercise intolerance. Closure of the large defect and surgical repair of associated abnormalities is always recommended. If large defects are left alone, permanent damage to the heart and lung vessels may occur in time, causing elevated pressure in the lungs or pulmonary hypertension. Diagnosis can be made accurately by ultrasonography (echo/Doppler, an ultrasonic picture of the heart). Diagnostic cardiac catheterization is required rarely to evaluate associated anomalies or complications such as pulmonary hypertension. Closure of uncomplicated small or moderate sized ostium secundum ASDs can often be accomplished non-surgically by closure devices delivered by a cardiac catheter (a hollow tube inserted into the heart) if there are adequate tissue margins around the defect determined by echocardiography. Otherwise, surgical closure of the defect, and when necessary, repair of the cleft mitral valve and rerouting of out-of-place (anomalous) pulmonary veins to the left atrium, will result in excellent and usually permanent repair with long life expectancy.

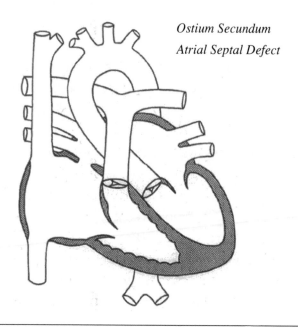

Ostium Secundum
Atrial Septal Defect

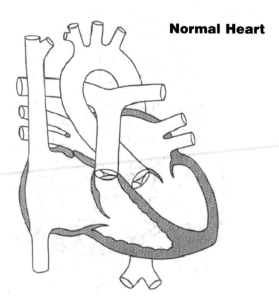

Normal Heart

Please refer to page 11 for a detailed illustration of the normal heart.

Atrioventricular Septal Defect (AVSD)

A complete *atrioventricular septal defect* (AVSD), also known as *endocardial cushion defect* or *complete or common atrioventricular canal,* involves a hole in the wall between both the upper and lower chambers of the heart and a malformation of the valves that divide the upper and lower chambers of the heart.

In a normal heart, the right and left heart chambers are completely separated by a solid wall called the septum. But a hole in the septum between the right and left upper chambers of the heart, called an atrial septal defect or ASD component, allows a stream of pink blood from the left atrium to cross over into the right atrium and to mix with the blue blood there. Consequently, an increased amount of blood flows through the right heart chambers and the pulmonary artery leading to the lungs. This added stream of fully oxygenated pink blood flowing through the lung vessels is a wasted effort as no further oxygen can be picked up. This ASD is of the ostium primum type.

In a child with AVSD, this condition is complicated by a second hole between the two lower pumping chambers (ventricles) of the heart, known as the ventricular septal defect or VSD component. This hole allows blood to cross from the left ventricle, where the pressure is high, into the right ventricle, where the pressure is much lower. The larger the hole, the more blood will cross from the left to the right side. The normal pressure in the left ventricle is much higher than in the right ventricle, so a significant amount of blood will cross through the hole unless it is quite small. This VSD is of the inlet muscular type.

The third aspect of AVSD is a malformation in the valves that divide the upper and lower chambers of the heart. Normally, there are two separate valves: a right-sided valve called the tricuspid valve, and a left-sided valve called the mitral valve. These two valves are often referred to as the atrioventricular valves because they separate the atria from the ventricles. Their normal function prevents blood from leaking back into the atria when the ventricles pump blood out of the heart to the lungs (from the right ventricle) and to the body (from the left ventricle). When the lower chambers are full, the atrioventricular valves are pushed shut and normally do not reopen until the ventricles are empty. With a complete AVSD, the tricuspid and mitral valves are not separated and work together as one common atrioventricular valve. These common atrioventricular valves almost always are regurgitant or leaky, adding additional volume strain on the heart.

When all three aspects of AVSD – ASD, VSD and valve regurgitation – are present as described above, a baby will probably show signs of congestive heart failure in the first months of life. Treatment with medications and diet will help until surgery is possible. Medications may include: digoxin, to help the heart cope with the increased workload; Lasix, to help the body remove excess water; and sometimes captopril, to help decrease the work of the heart. Higher calorie formula or powdered formula supplement to breast milk will help the baby gain weight. Rarely, the baby may require tube feedings to help with weight gain. Weight gain will make the baby a better surgical candidate with a lower post-operative complication rate.

AVSD requires open-heart surgery to close the two holes and separate the common valve into two valves. Surgery is often done between three and six months of age to allow the leaflets of the atrioventricular valve to thicken enough to hold a stitch better. After six months, there is a chance that lung damage can occur from the increased amount of blood that goes to the lung vessels. If for any reason the baby needs surgery earlier, the surgeon may perform a smaller operation to protect the baby's lungs until the total correction can proceed safely. This smaller surgery is called a pulmonary artery banding to prevent pulmonary overcirculation.

Some children have a less severe form of AVSD, called intermediate AVSD, in which one of the holes in either the upper or lower walls might be small or completely closed, or there might be a separation of the atrioventricular valves into nearly normal mitral and tricuspid valves. Children with intermediate AVSD will have milder symptoms than the child with complete AVSD, but will still require surgery to repair the defect.

Another variation of AVSD, called unbalanced AVSD, is complicated by blood flowing more toward one ventricle while the heart is still developing in the unborn baby. Uneven blood flow during heart development may result in one

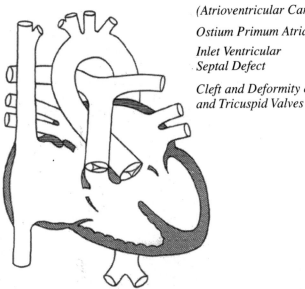

Endocardial Cushion Defect
(Atrioventricular Canal)
Ostium Primum Atrial Septal Defect
Inlet Ventricular
Septal Defect

Cleft and Deformity of Mitral
and Tricuspid Valves

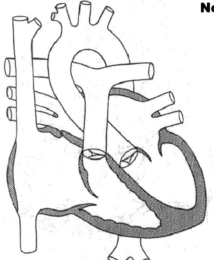

Normal Heart

Please refer to page 11 for a detailed
illustration of the normal heart.

ventricle being quite small. These babies cannot have the usual repair of AVSD, but will be treated as though the heart had only one pumping chamber. A pulmonary artery banding will be done in the first months of life to protect the lungs from too much blood flow. When the oxygen level of the baby drops as he outgrows the banding, usually between six and nine months of age, a bidirectional Glenn shunt may be done, followed by a Fontan procedure. (See chapter on Surgical Procedures for more information.)

AVSD is commonly seen in children with Down Syndrome. However, not all children with Down Syndrome have AVSD and not all children with AVSD have Down Syndrome.

Coarctation of the Aorta

The aorta is the largest blood vessel in the body. It is the passageway for the oxygen-rich pink arterial blood to leave the left side of the heart and deliver oxygen and nutrients to all parts of the body. It has three segments: the ascending aorta, the transverse aortic arch, and the descending aorta. When there is a narrowing in the aorta between the aortic arch and the descending aorta, this is called *coarctation of the aorta*. This defect can occur alone, isolated coarctation, or in combination with other heart defects.

Before birth, coarctation of the aorta is already present, but causes few if any problems because a large vessel, called the ductus arteriosus, effectively bridges the narrow area. The ductus is a blood vessel normally present in all unborn babies. It allows blood to bypass the lungs. After the baby begins to breathe air, the ductus closes off and ceases to function. Symptoms caused by coarctation can start very early in life after the ductus closes and turns into a fibrous cord or ligament. In rare cases, symptoms may not occur until adulthood.

Coarctation is characterized by high blood pressure in the upper body, especially the right arm, and weak pulses in the lower body, especially in the legs. If the narrowing is tight, symptoms can occur in the first days or weeks of life, since a tight coarctation creates extra work for the baby's heart pump, which may fail. Symptoms of heart failure include fast breathing, cough, chest congestion, poor weight gain, fast heart rate and poor feeding. If there are additional

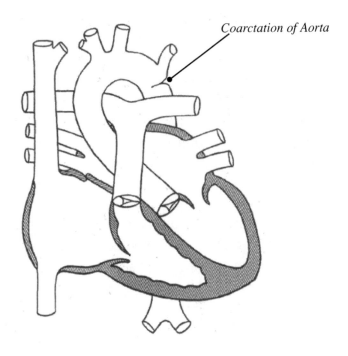

Coarctation of Aorta

Normal Heart

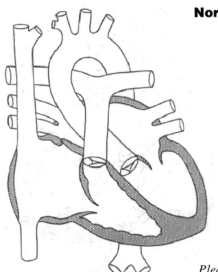

Please refer to page 11 for a detailed illustration of the normal heart.

heart defects, the symptoms may be more severe.

In older children and adults, coarctation may be detected when routine blood pressure measurement in the right arm reveals elevated blood pressure, or hypertension. Absence of pulses and/or low blood pressure in the legs confirms the presence of coarctation. Long standing hypertension damages the arteries in the upper body as well as the heart. Treatment is recommended as soon as the condition is recognized, regardless of symptoms, if right arm hypertension is present.

There are several options for treating coarctation of the aorta. In newborns with severe heart failure, temporary improvement can be achieved by a drug called prostaglandin. This drug allows the closed ductus arteriosus to reopen and temporarily bridge the narrowing. Surgical repair is done shortly after the baby's heart failure is brought under control. Most of the time, associated heart defects can be repaired during the same surgical procedure, but such a procedure would require open-heart surgery.

When there are no associated heart defects, repair of the coarctation is a closed-heart procedure. The surgical techniques have changed over time, but all aim at total removal of the narrow part of the aorta. Only rarely is a bypass graft required to bridge the narrowing. Current methods seldom require re-operation later in life. If further repair becomes necessary, non-surgical stretching, or dilation, of the narrow place can be accomplished by catheter balloon aortic angioplasty. In this procedure, a hollow balloon-tipped tube called a catheter is inserted into the aorta and the balloon is inflated to stretch the narrowing.

Coarctation repaired in early life can result in a lifelong cure. Long-standing high blood pressure, or hypertension, prior to repair, however, can permanently damage the arteries in the upper body so that even after repair, medication to lower blood pressure may be required daily. Prevention of subacute (slowly developing) bacterial endocarditis (SBE) prior to dental procedures needs to be observed both before and after coarctation repair. (See *Chapter Nine for more on SBE prophylaxis.*)

Congenitally Corrected Transposition of the Great Arteries

In *congenitally corrected transposition of the great arteries* (also called *ventricular inversion*), the aorta arises out of the right ventricle instead of the left ventricle, and the pulmonary artery comes off the left ventricle instead of the right ventricle. Normally, the right atrium connects to the right ventricle, which in turn connects to the pulmonary artery. On the left side of the heart, the left atrium connects to the left ventricle, which then connects to the aorta. With congenitally corrected transposition of the great arteries, the right atrium, which collects the blood as it returns from the body, depleted of oxygen, empties into the left ventricle instead of the right ventricle. The unoxygenated blood then empties through the mitral valve into the left ventricle, which connects to the pulmonary artery. The blood then flows to the lungs and returns to the left atrium through the pulmonary veins. The left atrium, instead of leading to the left ventricle, leads to the right ventricle through the tricuspid valve. The right ventricle directs the oxygenated blood out through the aorta to the rest of the body. The ventricles are inverted or transposed. **(A)** In about 20% of patients with congenitally corrected transposition of the great arteries, the heart is on the right side of the body, a condition known as dextrocardia.

With this defect, the blood is flowing through the lungs and body correctly, but by an abnormal path through the heart. The right ventricle, which normally pumps blood against low pressure to the lungs, pumps against the higher pressure of the body in a child with this defect. The child may not need surgery to correct the condition, but needs to be followed by a cardiologist. Because the right ventricle was not "built" to pump against higher pressure, the cardiologist watches to see that it continues to function properly, and that the tricuspid valve does not leak excessively. Patients with congenitally corrected transposition of the great arteries are also at risk for a problem with the heart's rhythm, known as complete heart block (CHB), in which the contractions of the upper and lower chambers of the heart are not in proper synchrony. The risk of CHB increases 12 % each year of life, even without surgery. Surgery increases the risk of developing CHB, necessitating pacemaker placement.

Congenitally Corrected Transposition of the Great Arteries and Ventricular Septal Defect

About 60% of the people with congenitally corrected transposition of the great arteries (see above) also have a hole in the wall, or septum, between the ventricles, called a *ventricular septal defect* (VSD). **(B)**

   • **Surgery**
   Ventricular septal defect requires surgical closure of the hole in the septum. This is usually done with a Gore-Tex patch sewn over the hole. It is open-heart surgery and the heart is stopped during the procedure. Since the electrical system of the heart runs along the septum, care is taken not to disturb this system, thus preventing heart rhythm changes. Patients with congenitally corrected transposition of the great arteries and ventricular septal defect are also at risk for developing complete heart block (CHB), as described above.

Congenitally Corrected Transposition of the Great Arteries, Ventricular Septal Defect and Pulmonary Stenosis or Atresia

About 30% of the patients with congenitally corrected transposition of the great arteries (see above) also have VSD and some type of obstruction to the flow of blood out of the left ventricle through the pulmonary valve. The valve is narrowed, or stenotic, or rarely it is closed completely, or atretic. This limits or prohibits blood from flowing out of the left ventricle to the lungs, forcing it through the VSD into the right ventricle. The baby will be blue or "cyanotic," because there is unoxygenated blood flowing out to the body. If the pulmonary stenosis is severe, medicine, such as prostaglandin, may be started as soon as the cardiologist has identified the defect. The medicine will be given intravenously to keep the patent ductus arteriosus open. Keeping this vessel open allows more oxygenated blood to flow to the body. **(C)**

   • **Surgery**
   In patients with severe pulmonary stenosis, the baby will be considered for a modified Blalock-Taussig shunt soon after birth. This is chest surgery, but not open-heart surgery, and the heart is not stopped. A Gore-Tex tube is place between the subclavian artery, the artery that runs under the collarbone, and the pulmonary artery. It is done either

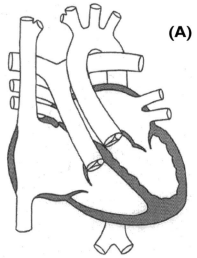

(A)

Ventricular Inversion
Transposition of the Great Arteries
Intact Ventricular Septum
Left Aortic Arch

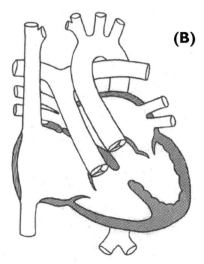

(B)

Ventricular Inversion
Transposition of the Great Arteries
Ventricular Septal Defect
Left Aortic Arch

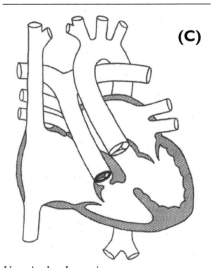

(C)

Ventricular Inversion
Transposition of the Great Arteries
Ventricular Septal Defect
Valvular and Subvalvular Pulmonary Stenosis
Left Aortic Arch

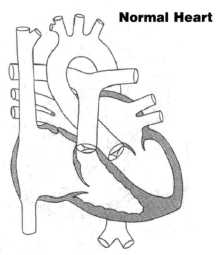

Normal Heart

Please refer to page 11 for a detailed
illustration of the normal heart.

through an incision over the baby's breastbone, or sternum, or through the baby's side, between the ribs. The shunt allows blood to flow from the baby's upper body directly to the lungs, not going through the heart at all. From the lungs, it flows to the heart to be pumped out to the body, carrying oxygen. This allows the baby to grow out of infancy with more oxygenated blood reaching the body. The blood flows through the pulmonary circulation, and allows the pulmonary arteries to grow better, in preparation for the next surgery.

When the child reaches two to four years of age, the repair surgery will be performed. First, the VSD will be closed by sewing a Gore-Tex patch over the hole. Then, a conduit will be placed from the left ventricle to the main pulmonary artery, thus bypassing the blockage near the pulmonary valve. This is open-heart surgery and the heart is stopped during the procedure. Since the electrical system of the heart runs along the septum, care is taken not to disturb this system, thus preventing heart rhythm changes. During this surgery, the modified Blalock-Taussig shunt is closed or "taken down." Patients with congenitally corrected transposition of the great arteries, ventricular septal defect and pulmonary stenosis or atresia are also at risk for developing complete heart block (CHB), as described above.

Since the right ventricle does not work well as the systemic pump over decades in the majority of patients, new surgical techniques for ventricular inversion are continuously being developed. One such recent surgical procedure is the double switch. In this procedure an atrial baffle is placed (venous switch) to divert the systemic veins to the left atrium and the pulmonary veins to the right atrium. In addition, an arterial switch is performed to switch the pulmonary artery and aorta and surgically correct the ventricular/great artery relationships. Thus, flow in these hearts after the double-switch are as follows: Systemic veins to left atrium to right ventricle to pulmonary artery, and also pulmonary veins to right atrium to left ventricle and then to the aorta. This is an extensive operation with higher surgical risk and potential for complications, such as complete heart block as noted above.

Double Inlet Left Ventricle (DILV)

Double inlet left ventricle (DILV) is the congenital heart defect most commonly referred to as "single ventricle." In the normal heart, the tricuspid valve allows oxygen-poor blue blood to flow from the right atrium to the right ventricle and then through the pulmonary artery to the lungs. The mitral valve allows oxygen-rich blood from the lungs to pass from the left atrium to the left ventricle and out to the body. But with DILV, both the tricuspid valve and the mitral valve lead into the left ventricle. The right ventricle is small and not well developed. There is a hole, called a ventricular septal defect (VSD), between these two chambers.

Double Inlet Left Ventricle with Pulmonary Stenosis

In this form of DILV, the pulmonary artery arises from the nonfunctional right ventricle and there is a "tightness" or stenosis of the pulmonary artery, causing less blood to get to the lungs. Because the unoxygenated blood enters the left ventricle and can flow to the aorta, the baby will be blue or "cyanotic."

• Surgery

The initial surgery will be a modified Blalock-Taussig (BT) shunt, connecting the subclavian artery to one of the pulmonary arteries. This allows more blood to get through the pulmonary arteries to the lungs. This allows the baby to be less cyanotic and allows the pulmonary arteries to grow in preparation for the next surgeries. The Blalock-Taussig shunt will be done in early infancy and will help the baby grow until later infancy (less than one year), at which time the Glenn procedure is performed.

The Glenn procedure connects the superior vena cava (SVC) to the pulmonary artery, after the BT shunt is separated. This allows even more blood flow through the pulmonary arteries to the lungs. It also serves as a basis for the final surgery, the Fontan procedure.

The Fontan procedure takes the blood through the inferior vena cava (IVC), directly to the pulmonary arteries with the SVC blood. All the blood then goes to the lungs for oxygenation before going to the heart for pumping to the body.

Double Inlet Left Ventricle without Pulmonary Stenosis

In this form of DILV, there is no narrowing below the pulmonary valve and the pulmonary valve itself is normal. Thus the patient will develop excessive pulmonary blood flow soon after birth.

• **Surgery**

A pulmonary artery band is placed surgically to decrease the amount of pulmonary blood flow. Later in the first year of life, the band is removed and a Glenn shunt is performed. When the patient is between 2 and 4 years of age, the Fontan procedure is then performed as outlined above.

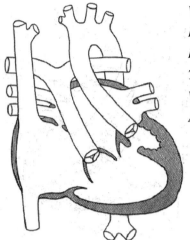

Ventricular Inversion

Double-inlet Left Ventricle

Rudimentary Right Ventricle (outlet chamber)

Transposition of the Great Arteries

Ventricular Septal Defect (outlet foramen)

Atrial Septal Defect

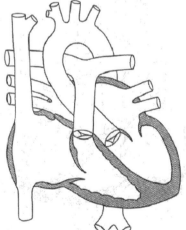

Normal Heart

Please refer to page 11 for a detailed illustration of the normal heart.

Double Outlet Right Ventricle (DORV)

With the defect known as *double outlet right ventricle* (DORV), which accounts for less than 1% of all congenital heart defects, both of the heart's "outlets," the aorta and the pulmonary artery, arise from the right ventricle. In the normal heart, the aorta arises from the left ventricle and the pulmonary artery arises from the right ventricle. DORV is usually accompanied by a large ventricular septal defect (VSD), which serves as the outlet for blood from the left ventricle. While the relationship of the aorta and the pulmonary artery plus the position of the VSD vary greatly with different forms of this defect, they are crucial in diagnosis and plan of treatment.

DORV: Subaortic Ventricular Septal Defect with Side-by-Side Position of the Great Arteries (Aorta/Pulmonary Artery)

When the VSD lies closest to the aortic valve, it is called "subaortic." This is the most common form of DORV, accounting for 60-70% of all DORVs. The aorta lies to the right of the pulmonary artery and the VSD is below or near the aortic valve. Blood comes from the body into the heart through the right atrium, then crosses the tricuspid valve and enters the right ventricle. It then flows out to the pulmonary artery or the aorta. It continues through the pulmonary artery, to the lungs and back to the left side of the heart. After flowing through the left atrium and left ventricle, it flows through the VSD, the only way out of the left ventricle. Since the VSD is directly below the aorta, the blood then continues up the aorta.

• Surgery

A tunnel is created from the left ventricle through the VSD toward the aorta. This prevents unoxygenated blood from entering the aorta and traveling to the body, and allows it to travel only to the lungs. From the lungs, it flows to the left side of the heart through this tunnel then out the aorta to the body. This procedure can be done by the time the child reaches six months of age.

DORV: Subaortic Ventricular Septal Defect with Side-by-Side Position of the Great Arteries (Aorta/Pulmonary Artery) and Pulmonary Stenosis (Fallot type)

In about 50% of patients with this form of DORV, pulmonary stenosis also occurs. In this combination, blood comes from the body into the heart through the right atrium and into the right ventricle. Because the pulmonary valve is stenotic or "tight," most of the blood flows through the aorta instead of going out the pulmonary artery to the lungs for oxygen. This means unoxygenated blood goes back to the body. The small amount of blood that goes to the lungs comes back to the left side of the heart. After flowing through the left atrium and left ventricle, it flows through the VSD, the only way out of the left ventricle. Since the VSD is directly below the aorta, the blood then continues up the aorta. Because most of the unoxygenated blood goes to the body, the baby will be blue or "cyanotic." This is similar to another defect called "tetralogy of Fallot," in which a VSD and pulmonary stenosis are two of the four components. That is why this may be referred to as a "Fallot type" defect. **(A)**

• **Surgery**

A tunnel is surgically created from the left ventricle through the VSD to the aorta. This prevents the unoxygenated blood from the right ventricle from traveling through the aorta to the body. Blood from the right ventricle can only go out the pulmonary artery, so the pulmonary stenosis must be relieved. The tight area of the valve may be able to be opened. If possible, the surgeon will open the valve or place a "patch" to enlarge the area. The surgery is done anywhere between 6 months to 2 years of age.

Occasionally, the pulmonary valve cannot be repaired, and a Blalock Taussig shunt is surgically placed during early infancy, if the child is very blue. This surgery allows some blood to get to the lungs, decreasing cyanosis temporarily and allowing the pulmonary arteries to grow. Then, corrective repair can be undertaken when the child outgrows the size of the shunt and becomes more cyanotic (usually within the first 5 years of life).

A "conduit" or tube containing another valve can then be surgically placed on the outside of the heart. This tube is attached at one end to the right ventricle and to the pulmonary artery at the other end, bypassing the stenotic area. By delaying this surgery until the child is closer to 5 years of age, placement of a larger conduit, adequate for the child to grow, is possible. This delays and helps prevent future procedures.

Subpulmonic Ventricular Septal Defect with Side-by-Side Position of the Great Arteries (Aorta/Pulmonary Artery) (Taussig-Bing type)

This type of DORV is rare, accounting for approximately 8 to 10% of all DORVs. It is very similar to the defect known as transposition of the great arteries. The blood returning to the heart from the body enters the right atrium and then the right ventricle and heads out the aorta, taking unoxygenated blood back to the body. Blood coming back to the left side of the heart from the lungs passes out of the VSD up the pulmonary artery and back to the lungs. **(B)**

• Surgery

If the PDA closes soon after birth and the ASD is small or "restrictive," the newborn may need to go to the cardiac catheterization laboratory soon after birth to have a Rashkind procedure, or balloon septostomy, completed. This is not surgery. Through a small tube threaded through the infant's leg up into the heart, a deflated balloon is guided to the left atrium, inflated and pulled through the ASD to "stretch" it to a larger size. Enlarging the ASD in this fashion allows the baby to receive more oxygenated blood to the body. During the cardiac catheterization, the cardiologist will take more pictures with dye, or angiograms, to help identify the specifics of the baby's heart. The Rashkind procedure is most effective in the newborn period, when the septal wall is most likely to stretch well. After that, the older infant may need surgery to create or enlarge the ASD, if corrective surgery needs to be delayed.

With this condition, the baby is blue because mostly unoxygenated blood is recirculating through the body. Surgical intervention, therefore, must be done early, by 3 to 4 months of age. An Arterial Switch operation is usually the preferred procedure. It is open-heart surgery and the heart is stopped during the surgery. The aorta is cut above the level of the coronary arteries. The pulmonary artery is cut at the same level. The coronary arteries are removed from the remaining base of the aorta and then reattached to the base of the pulmonary artery. Then the aorta is sewn to the base of the pulmonary artery and the pulmonary artery is sewn to the base of the aorta, essentially switching the circulation and

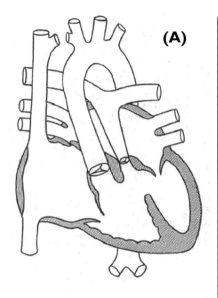

(A)

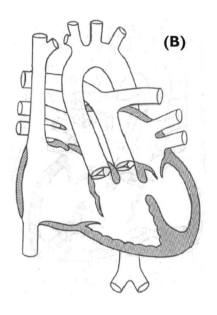

(B)

Double-Outlet Right Ventricle
Side-by-Side Great Arteries
Pulmonary Stenosis
Ventricular Septal Defect

Double-Outlet Right Ventricle
Transposed Great Arteries
Ventricular Septal Defect

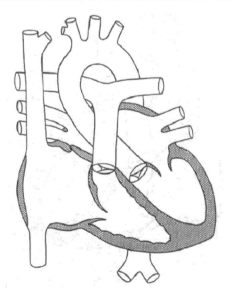

Normal Heart

Please refer to page 11
for a detailed illustration
of the normal heart.

preserving the coronary circulation. Along with the arterial switch, an intraventricular tunnel is created between the left ventricle and the new aorta to effectively close the VSD. The pulmonary artery now comes off the right ventricle, ready to carry the blood to the lungs for oxygen.

Ebstein's Malformation

Ebstein's Malformation is an abnormality of the tricuspid valve, the valve that allows blood to pass from the right atrium into the right ventricle. When the three leaflets that comprise this valve close properly, blood is forced to the lungs whenever the ventricle contracts. But if the tricuspid valve does not close properly, blood can leak back into the right atrium. With Ebstein's Malformation, the leaflets are improperly located, which often prevents them from coming together to form a tight seal.

In addition, most children with Ebstein's Malformation also have a hole between the right and left atria, called an atrial septal defect. When the tricuspid valve is leaky and the right ventricle does not pump properly, oxygen-poor blue blood will cross through the atrial hole and mix with the oxygen-rich blood in the left side of the heart. Babies with this condition may be noticeably blue shortly after birth and show signs of heart failure, including fast breathing, fast heart rate and poor circulation. In severe forms of Ebstein's Malformation, the leaflets may be far displaced into the right ventricle, causing the ventricle to be less muscular and therefore to pump less effectively.

Surgery to repair severe cases of Ebstein's Malformation and close the atrial septal defect, if present, may need to be done. Repair requires open-heart surgery. The surgeon may be able to relocate the abnormal leaflet or may need to replace the entire valve. If replacement is necessary, a tissue valve from a pig or cow, called a bioprosthesis, is used. If the right ventricle is unable to pump normally because of abnormal muscle development, additional surgery similar to that done for tricuspid atresia will also be required. In milder forms of Ebstein's Malformation, a child may be observed for signs of deteriorating valve function for years or decades before surgery is required.

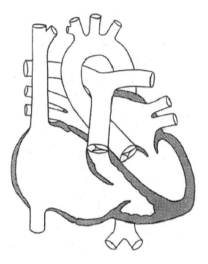

*Ebstein's Malformation
of Tricuspid Valve*

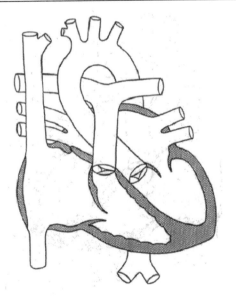

Normal Heart

*Please refer to page 11
for a detailed illustration
of the normal heart.*

Hypoplastic Left Heart Syndrome (HLHS)

Hypoplastic left heart syndrome (HLHS) occurs in about 1% of all congenital heart disease cases. The left ventricle (LV) is hypoplastic, meaning it is under-developed or not functioning. Essentially, the LV is not functional because the valves leading into and out of the LV, the mitral and aortic valves, are severely stenosed (tight), or atretic, meaning impassable or not allowing any blood flow. In addition, the main route out of the left ventricle, the aorta, is also hypoplastic. The newborn baby may initially appear to be well during the first hours or even days of life. However, as the baby breathes on his own, the pressure in his lungs begins to decrease. Also, the patent ductus arteriosus, a tiny vessel between the aorta and pulmonary artery, will begin to close after birth. Then, the baby will appear sicker, breathing quickly, not feeding, showing a faster heart beat and congested lungs.

Initially, the cardiologist may order intravenous medication, prostaglandin E1, to be given to keep the patent ductus arteriosus open. During this time, the baby may have to have a breathing tube in place. The effects of prostaglandins on the ductus is limited as the patient usually develops tolerance to the medication over the first few weeks of life.

• Surgery

Within days or hours after a definitive diagnosis is formed, the baby will go for the first surgery, called a Norwood procedure. The pulmonary artery is separated from the heart and connected to the small aorta. This enlarges the aorta and allows both oxygenated and deoxygenated blood to get to the body via the open pulmonary valve. Additionally, a modified Blalock-Taussig shunt, or a valveless conduit from the right ventricle to the pulmonary artery (Sano modification), is placed. In the modified Blalock-Taussig shunt, a Gore-Tex tube is placed between the subclavian artery, the artery that runs under the collar bone, and the pulmonary artery to allow blood to flow from the baby's upper body directly to the lungs, bypassing the heart altogether. From the lungs, blood flows to the heart to be pumped out to the body, carrying oxygen. This allows the baby to grow out of infancy with more oxygenated blood reaching the body. The blood flow through the pulmonary circulation allows the

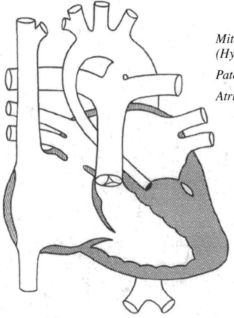

*Mitral-Aortic Valve Atresia
(Hypoplastic left heart)*

Patent Ductus Arteriosus

Atrial Septal Defect

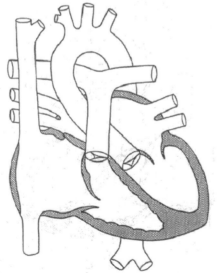

Normal Heart

*Please refer to page 11
for a detailed illustration
of the normal heart.*

pulmonary arteries to grow better, in preparation for the next surgery, which will be at four to eight months of age.

At this time, the Glenn procedure is performed. The Glenn procedure connects the superior vena cava (SVC) to the pulmonary artery, after the BT shunt is separated. This allows even more blood flow through the pulmonary arteries to the lungs. It also serves as a basis for the final surgery, the Fontan procedure. The Fontan procedure takes the blood through the inferior vena cava (IVC), directly to the pulmonary arteries with the SVC blood. All the blood then goes to the lungs for oxygenation before going to the heart for pumping to the body.

In an attempt to diminish the mortality and morbidity of the modified Norwood procedure, a new combined cardiac catheterization and surgical approach called the hybrid procedure has been developed. In the hybrid procedure, a catheterization is performed and a stent is placed in the patent ductus arteriosus to maintain its patency. A balloon atrial septostomy is also performed if the hole in the atrial septum is restrictive to blood flow. Then a limited closed surgical procedure is performed to band the branch pulmonary arteries to prevent excessive pulmonary blood flow. The Glenn procedure is then performed at 4-8 months of age, where the pulmonary artery bands are removed and aortic arch reconstruction is performed, if necessary. Finally, the Fontan procedure is done between 2-4 years of age.

Mitral Valve Abnormalities

The mitral valve is on the left side of the heart, between the left atrium (LA) and the left ventricle (LV). The left atrium receives oxygenated blood from the lungs. Blood passes through the mitral valve to the left ventricle to be pumped out to the body.

Mitral Valve Stenosis

Stenosis is a tightening or narrowing of the valve. Because the valve is constricted, blood cannot easily get through it to the left ventricle. As a result, blood backs up in the left atrium causing the LA to enlarge. This, in turn, causes further backup of blood in the lungs, which may cause difficulty breathing. The increased blood in the lungs may elevate the lung pressure, called pulmonary hypertension. Without intervention, the right side of the heart can also become enlarged trying to pump blood to the already saturated lungs.

Relief of the stenosis is necessary to prevent irreversible damage to the heart and lungs. Balloon valvuloplasty may be successful in relieving mitral valve stenosis. In this procedure, done in the cardiac catheterization laboratory, a catheter tube is inserted through the groin and moved up into the heart. The tube crosses the mitral valve, where a very tiny balloon is inflated at the tip of a special catheter. The balloon is then pulled through the mitral valve, stretching the valve open. There is a risk of the valve leaking after this procedure, because of the stretching. This balloon procedure has been performed primarily in patients with mitral stenosis after rheumatic heart disease.

More often, and with greater success, mitral valve stenosis is relieved with a mitral valve repair. This is open-heart surgery. Occasionally, if the valve is not repairable, a mitral valve replacement surgery is required to correct the condition.

Mitral Valve Regurgitation

Normally, the mitral valve functions like a gate, closing tightly once the LA empties and the LV is full, allowing no blood to leak back into the LA. In *mitral valve regurgitation,* sometimes referred to as *mitral insufficiency,* the mitral valve does not close well and blood leaks back into the LA. This causes the LA to dilate, or enlarge. This insufficiency of the mitral valve can also occur as a complication of rheumatic fever. Depending on its severity, mitral valve regurgitation can be treated with medication. Mitral valve regurgitation and its subsequent LA enlargement may lead to arrhythmias. Medications may include drugs that help control these abnormal heart rhythms.

When mitral valve regurgitation does not respond to the necessary medications, surgical correction is necessary. Mitral valve repair and mitral valve replacement are the two open-heart surgical options to repair the mitral valve. Recently, new cardiac catheterization techniques are being developed to install clips on the mitral valve to diminish the amount of leaking.

Mitral Valve Prolapse

Normally, the two leaflets of the mitral valve close tightly once the LA empties and the LV is full, allowing no blood to leak back into the LA. In *mitral valve
prolapse*, one of the leaflets extends back into the LA, or prolapses, instead of
stopping even with its attachment to the annulus, or ring, of the valve.

This is a very common defect. It is estimated that 5% of the entire population
has mitral valve prolapse. It is most commonly diagnosed in adolescence and
early adulthood. Mitral valve prolapse can be developmental in the majority
of patients. This means that the valve may cease to prolapse as one's connec-
tive tissue gets stiffer as one ages into adulthood. Most people require no
treatment.

Mitral Valve Insufficiency

Cleft Mitral Valve With Intact Atrial Septum

Gigantic Left Atrium

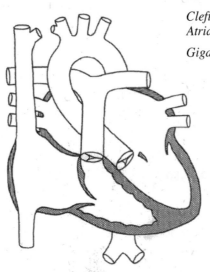

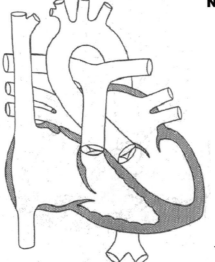

Normal Heart

Please refer to page 11 for a detailed illustration of the normal heart.

Patent Ductus Arteriosus (PDA)

The *patent ductus arteriosus* (PDA) is a blood vessel normally present in all unborn babies connecting the pulmonary artery and the aorta. It allows blood to bypass the lungs and go directly out to the body because in the fetus the lungs are not providing oxygen to the baby. The baby's oxygen supply comes from the mother's placenta until the baby is born. After birth, when the baby breathes air, the PDA normally closes within a few hours or days.

In some cases, however, the PDA remains open, or patent. The chances of this happening are much higher in premature infants due to a lack of mature muscle tone in the wall of this blood vessel. Sometimes, the PDA may only partially close.

If the PDA does not close after birth, blood from the aorta will flow back through the PDA into the lung vessels, producing a heart murmur. This might be the only sign that the child has a heart defect. Some premature babies with a large PDA, however, may be quite sick, requiring special medication or surgical treatment.

When a baby has other heart defects, especially complex defects, it is not uncommon for the PDA to stay open. The diagnosis of PDA is confirmed by doing an echocardiogram. Usually no further testing is required. If a PDA stays open beyond the newborn period, the chance of spontaneous closure is small.

Depending on the size and length of the PDA, it may be able to be closed by a coiling procedure or placement of an occluder plug done in the cardiac catheterization lab. Small coils or an occluder plug are placed in the PDA though a catheter that is threaded to the heart through a large vessel. The coil or plug will cause the PDA to clot and close. (See *Chapter Four, under Cardiac Catheterization, for more information.*)

For premature infants who are not candidates for the coiling procedure, a medication called indomethacin may be effective in closing the PDA. If the medication does not work or cannot be given due to risk of complication, surgery may be required.

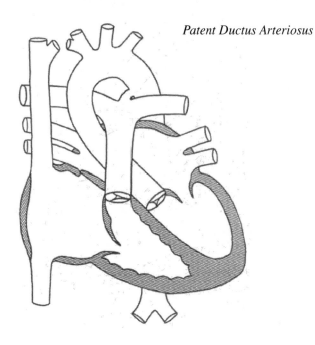

Patent Ductus Arteriosus

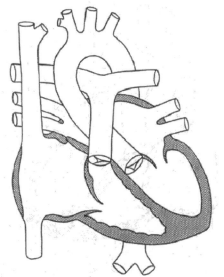

Normal Heart

*Please refer to page 11
for a detailed illustration
of the normal heart.*

Pulmonary Atresia with Intact Ventricular Septum

The term *pulmonary atresia* means that there is no exit for the blood to be pumped out from the right ventricle into the pulmonary artery. When there is no associated ventricular septal defect, or hole in the right ventricle, the right ventricle cannot fill normally and usually remains very small. This heart condition is sometimes referred to as *hypoplastic right ventricle complex.*

When the right ventricle pumps, the blood cannot exit and the pressure within the ventricle becomes extremely high. This high pressure forces some of the blood through the tricuspid valve back into the right upper chamber, a condition known as tricuspid regurgitation. A naturally occurring opening in the wall of the right upper chamber, the right atrium, called the foramen ovale, allows a stream of blue blood to cross over to the pink-blooded left upper chamber, the left atrium, and then to the left pumping chamber, the left ventricle, and out to the aorta. The lung circulation is supplied by means of the ductus arteriosus. The mixed blue and pink blood in the aorta gives the infant a bluish discoloration, called cyanosis.

In this form of pulmonary atresia, the right ventricle is small and muscle bound. The tricuspid valve, which separates the right atrium from the right ventricle, can be abnormally small as well. Even during fetal life, the blood trapped in the right ventricle seeks to get out each time the heart pumps, during the part of the pulse called systole. Some blood will leak out through the tricuspid valve, but the high pressure in the ventricle can also force the blood through openings in the right ventricular heart muscle itself, called sinusoids, that eventually enter the coronary circulation. These coronary sinusoids can become a problem when the high pressure in the right ventricle is surgically lowered.

Infants born with this condition require immediate cardiac care. If left alone, the patent or open ductus arteriosus (PDA) will close in the first hours or days of life. The PDA must be kept open with the help of medication called prostaglandin. Occasionally, a restrictive opening in the atrial wall, called the foramen ovale, must be enlarged with a balloon catheter to allow free blood flow from right to left atrium.

Recently, noninvasive cardiac catheterization techniques have been developed in patients with pulmonary atresia with intact ventricular septum that have a

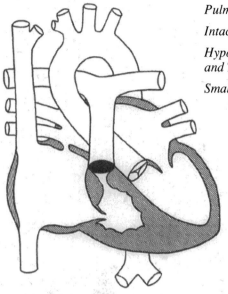

Pulmonary Valve Atresia

Intact Ventricular Septum

Hypoplastic Right Ventricle and Tricuspid Valve

Small Atrial Septal Defect

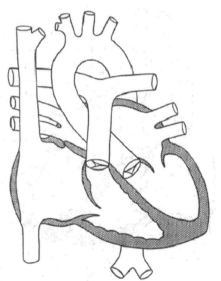

Normal Heart

Please refer to page 11 for a detailed illustration of the normal heart.

right ventricular size that is sufficient. Laser or radiofrequency pulmonary val-
votomy can be performed with special catheters as well as ballooning open
a small atrial connection.

The extent of the emergency operation that will follow depends on the nature of pulmonary atresia. Most patients will require a shunt operation to
replace the precarious PDA. A plastic tube is placed surgically between the
aorta and the pulmonary artery to provide steady blood flow for lung circulation. This is called a modified Blalock-Taussig shunt. If there is a fused pulmonary valve, the valve is opened to allow the ventricle to function.

When corrective surgery is considered in older infants and children, there
are several options, depending on the condition of the right ventricle. A two-
ventricle repair can be accomplished in those patients in whom the right ventricle and pulmonary artery have grown to the point that they can support
the right heart circulation.

In patients where the right ventricle remains small, a one-and-one-half ventricle repair can be considered. This is similar to the two-ventricle repair except that it requires an additional bi-directional cavo-pulmonary shunt, called
a Glenn shunt. Glenn shunt is a connection between the superior vena cava
and the pulmonary arteries that enables half of the oxygen-poor blue blood
to reach the pulmonary arteries without passing through the small ventricle.

In those patients where the right ventricle is tiny, or especially if there are
coronary sinusoids, the one-ventricle repair, called the Fontan operation, is the
remaining surgical option.

All the blue blood in the right atrium is channeled directly to the pulmonary
arteries, completely bypassing the right ventricle. Although a heart with only a
single functioning ventricle is not as effective as one with two ventricles, persons
with Fontan repair can enjoy a productive life well into adulthood. Patients with
Fontan operation require regular checkups by a cardiologist, often require anticoagulants, and must observe SBE (subacute bacterial endocarditis) prophylaxis
prior to dental procedures. (See Chapter Nine for more on SBE prophylaxis.)

Pulmonary Atresia with Ventricular Septal Defect (VSD)

The term *pulmonary atresia* means there is no opening for blood to exit from the right ventricle into the pulmonary artery. Normally, there is a pulmonic valve that opens and allows blood to exit the heart through the right ventricle. In pulmonary atresia, however, the valve is permanently sealed or absent. The main pulmonary artery (or pulmonary trunk) is either small, string-like, or completely absent. Pulmonary atresia takes one of two forms: with or without ventricular septal defect (VSD).

The associated ventricular septal defect is a large hole in the wall that separates the two ventricles and allows the blue right-ventricular blood to pass through to the left ventricle and out to the aorta. This condition is closely related to tetralogy of Fallot. It is sometimes called pseudotruncus because of its similarity to truncus arteriosus, in which there is only one vessel emerging from the heart. Since blood required for lung circulation cannot come from the right ventricle, survival depends on the existence of alternative routes. A ductus arteriosus brings blood from the aorta to the pulmonary artery, or if the ductus is absent, multiple large collateral (bypass) arteries known as MAPCAs emerge from the aorta and supply the lung circulation with blood.

In this defect, the blood in the aorta is a mixture of blue and pink blood from the two ventricles that give the child a bluish discoloration, called cyanosis. This purple blood is pumped to the body and also reaches the lung vessels by means of a ductus arteriosus or MAPCAs. A newborn with severe cyanosis may receive a medication called prostaglandin to keep the ductus temporarily open. Nevertheless, a newborn with pulmonary atresia will seldom be discharged without first undergoing a surgical procedure to provide a more reliable blood flow to the lungs. A preoperative cardiac catheterization is often recommended to define the size of lung vessels and the source of blood supply.

Surgery at this early age is called palliative, or supportive surgery. Corrective open-heart surgery is usually recommended at a later date. The palliative procedure for young infants involves insertion of a shunt, a small plastic tube, between the pulmonary artery and the aorta. The shunt has the same role as the naturally occurring ductus arteriosus: it supplies the lung circulation with blood.

Some infants may require a second shunt surgery on the opposite side of the chest if the oxygen content in the aortic blood remains low, causing the blood to appear to be too blue, or if the branch pulmonary arteries fail to grow to a size that allows complete repair of this heart defect.

An infant born dependent on MAPCAs for pulmonary blood flow will require several palliative operations to prepare for the ultimate corrective surgery. These MAPCAs are multiple disconnected arteries, each feeding a separate part of the lungs. They must be joined together, a process called unifocalization, to form a single right and left branch pulmonary artery. After this is successfully accomplished, corrective surgery may follow.

All patients with pulmonary atresia undergoing corrective surgery will require substitution for the missing main pulmonary artery. This open-heart procedure, known as the Rastelli operation, consists of closing the VSD with a large plastic patch and placing a new pulmonary artery between the right ventricle and the branch pulmonary arteries. This new artery can be a prosthetic valved conduit made of plastic or a homograft harvested from human cadaver tissue.

This prosthetic valved conduit substitutes for the pulmonary artery. It cannot grow as the child gets older and bigger. Thus, it will have to be replaced when it becomes obstructive. It is estimated that a toddler undergoing the Rastelli operation will require several operations throughout his or her lifetime. One should keep in mind, however, that for a child born with a major cardiac malformation and an uncertain future, a successful Rastelli operation provides a near normal existence well into adult life.

All patients who have had cardiac repair using foreign material, such as shunts, conduits, patches or valves, must observe SBE precautions. (*See Chapter Nine for more on SBE prophylaxis.*) Some patients will also require blood clot prevention medicines, such as aspirin or Coumadin.

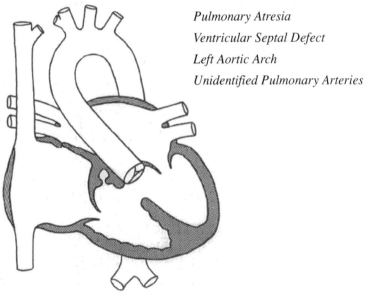

Pulmonary Atresia
Ventricular Septal Defect
Left Aortic Arch
Unidentified Pulmonary Arteries

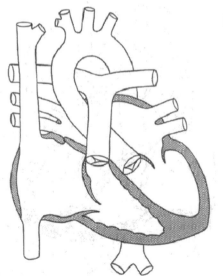

Normal Heart

Please refer to page 11
for a detailed illustration
of the normal heart.

Pulmonary Stenosis

Pulmonary stenosis is a narrowing or obstruction between the right ventricle and the pulmonary (lung) circulation. It is frequently associated with other anomalies, although here we will look at pulmonary stenosis as an isolated abnormality. The obstruction can occur at several levels:

- The most common obstruction is the pulmonary valve stenosis. A normal pulmonary valve allows blood to flow freely from the heart's pumping chamber, the right ventricle, into the vessels leading to the lungs, the pulmonary arteries. The valve usually has three leaflets, or cusps, that open widely when the ventricle pumps. When the ventricle relaxes, the leaflets close tightly and do not allow backflow, or regurgitation, of blood into the right ventricle from the pulmonary artery. In valvar stenosis, the leaflets are partially fused together and unable to open completely. Frequently, there are only two leaflets, called a bicuspid valve, instead of three. Pulmonary valve stenosis creates extra work for the right ventricle that must deliver the blood into the pulmonary arteries regardless of how tight the narrowing. Heart failure occurs when the ventricle can no longer deliver.

- Part of the right ventricle below the pulmonary valve is called the outflow tract of the right ventricle. This muscular tunnel (infundibulum) just below the valve is normally unobstructed and participates in pumping action. An abnormally thickened outflow muscle can narrow the tunnel resulting in subvalvar (or subpulmonic or infundibular) stenosis.

- A narrowing that occurs in the body of the right ventricle due to an abnormal muscle bundle is called a divided or double-chambered right ventricle.

- A narrowing of the pulmonary artery after it branches off to the left and right lung is called branch pulmonary artery stenosis, or peripheral pulmonary artery stenosis. A narrowing of the main pulmonary trunk just above the valve is called supravalvar pulmonic stenosis.

Regardless of the area where pulmonary stenosis occurs (below the valve, at the valve, above the valve, or in any combination), the end result is increased work for

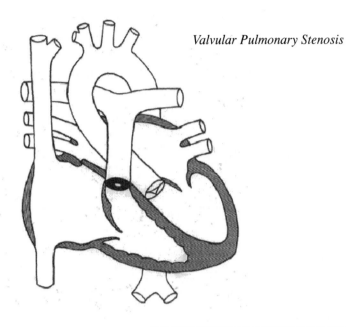

Valvular Pulmonary Stenosis

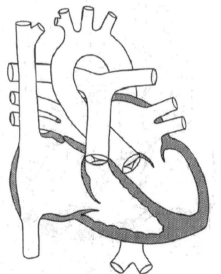

Normal Heart

*Please refer to page 11
for a detailed illustration
of the normal heart.*

the right ventricle. Unless the stenosis is very severe in infancy, there are often few symptoms. The only clue may be the presence of a loud heart murmur.

Newborns with severe or critical pulmonic stenosis can become very ill shortly after birth with congestive heart failure and cyanosis (blue discoloration) and require urgent treatment by surgery or by catheter balloon valvuloplasty.

Very mild forms of pulmonary stenosis may not require treatment, but a growing child must be watched for progression of narrowing by regular visits to the cardiologist, with periodic echocardiographic monitoring.

When the stenosis is severe enough to require treatment, there are several options, depending on the area of stenosis. Stenosis that involves fusion of the valve leaflets (pulmonary valvar stenosis) can often be treated by balloon valvuloplasty during cardiac catheterization. A special hollow plastic tube with an inflatable balloon at the tip is inserted in a large vein in the groin. This catheter is advanced into the right ventricle and further across the pulmonary valve narrowing where it is positioned between the fused valve leaflets. The balloon is then filled with fluid, which causes the fused leaflets to separate and open. This procedure is done under heavy sedation, and may require an overnight stay in the hospital. If the narrowing recurs, repeated valvuloplasty can be performed, or the patient may be referred to surgery.

When the obstruction is below or above the valve, surgery is the choice for repair. The operation requires open-heart surgery and the use of a heart-lung bypass machine. While work is done inside the heart, the machine maintains the patient's circulation. If there is obstructive muscle in the ventricle, it is removed. If there is a "waist" in the pulmonary artery above the valve, it is enlarged with a patch. If valve leaflets are fused, they are opened.

Peripheral pulmonary arteries can be repaired surgically by patching the narrow vessels, but recurrence of such narrowing is not unusual. An alternative treatment is catheter balloon dilation, which stretches the arteries. Once the arteries are enlarged, one or more rigid tubes, or intravascular stents, may be placed inside the vessels to keep them permanently open.

With the exception of very sick infants, the in-hospital recovery time is often just a few days. Mild narrowings that may be left after treatment are well tolerated, requiring minimal or no lifestyle restrictions.

Tetralogy of Fallot (TOF)

Tetralogy of Fallot (TOF) is a combination of four different heart problems. The term "tetralogy" comes from the Greek word for "four." The four problems are: pulmonary stenosis (PS), ventricular septal defect (VSD), overriding of the aorta, and right ventricular hypertrophy. It is helpful to first understand each of the four defects separately and then look at the effect of their combination on the heart.

Pulmonary Stenosis

When the pulmonary artery, the artery that carries blue blood from the right ventricle to the lungs, is blocked, the condition is called pulmonary stenosis. The blockage may be the result of too much muscle below the pulmonary valve or that the valve itself is too small or unable to open all the way. The blood vessel, the main pulmonary artery, also may be too narrow above the valve. In severe cases of TOF, the entire pulmonary arterial system can be underdeveloped with all branches being smaller than normal. This condition is called hypoplastic pulmonary arteries.

Ventricular Septal Defect

A ventricular septal defect (VSD) is a hole between the two lower pumping chambers (ventricles) of the heart. This is the most common of all congenital heart defects. In TOF, the hole is very large and situated under the aorta. The pressure in the two ventricles is equally high due to the large hole.

Overriding Aorta

Normally the aorta comes from the left lower chamber of the heart, the left ventricle. The aorta is the largest blood vessel in the heart and carries pink blood from the heart to all parts of the body. When the aorta is described as overriding, it means that the vessel is inappropriately positioned and straddles both the right and left ventricle just above the ventricular septal defect.

Right Ventricular Hypertrophy

The right ventricle is the lower chamber of the heart that pumps blue blood to the pulmonary arteries. Normally, the RV muscle is thin. Hypertrophy means the muscle wall of the chamber has become thickened. This occurs in TOF because of the extra work the muscle must do to pump blood past the blocked pulmonary artery as well as pump blood to the high-pressure aorta.

The combination of these four heart defects comprises the condition called tetralogy of Fallot. The result is that blue blood from the right ventricle is partially blocked from getting to the lungs. Instead, some blood can go through the VSD and out the overriding aorta to the body. The more severe the blockage in the pulmonary arteries, the more blue blood will go out the aorta instead. When blue blood goes out to the body, the child will not appear as pink as normal; his or her skin, lips and nails will appear to have a bluish color. This is called cyanosis.

The severity of pulmonary stenosis in TOF can vary quite a bit. It may be very mild in the newborn because very little blue blood will go out the aorta. The pulmonary stenosis, however, tends to become more severe as the baby grows. The baby's oxygen level will slowly decrease, until surgical correction of the TOF will become necessary. If the branches of the pulmonary artery are close to normal size, this operation can be done in one step.

If, however, the pulmonary arteries of the baby are hypoplastic, that is, too small, an additional procedure may be needed first to help these blood vessels grow to a more normal size. This operation, usually done in the first months of life, involves creating a shunt to force more blood into the pulmonary arteries, causing them to grow over time while bringing more blood to the lungs and raising the baby's oxygen level.

Complete repair of TOF is usually done in the first year of life. Complete repair of TOF consists of patch closure of the VSD so that the aorta arises solely from the LV, as well as enlarging the RV outflow tract, pulmonary valve, and branch PAs as much as possible. A severe event called a "tet spell" can be seen in children with severe tetralogy of Fallot, especially if the child has a

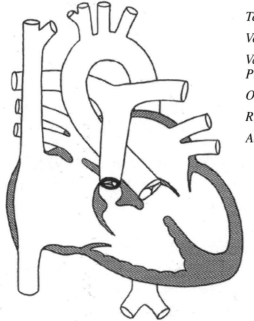

Tetralogy of Fallot

Ventricular Septal Defect

Valvular & Infundibular Pulmonary Stenosis

Overriding Aorta

Right Ventricular Hypertrophy

Atrial Septal Defect

Normal Heart

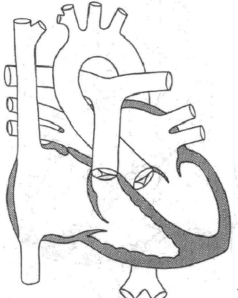

Please refer to page 11 for a detailed illustration of the normal heart.

great deal of extra muscle in the right ventricle blocking the area below the pulmonary artery. In a "tet spell," the extra muscle in the heart below the pulmonary valve may squeeze down tightly, allowing very little blood to get to the lungs. The baby will become irritable and very blue, breath very fast and may even pass out. If this happens, bring the baby's knees all the way up to his chest, call 911 and alert the doctor immediately. A "tet spell" can be very dangerous for the baby and may require urgent surgery. There are also medications that can be used to treat a "tet spell," or prevent it from occurring again.

Total Anomalous Pulmonary Venous Return (TAPVR)

When the heart and lungs are developing in the fetus, four veins will grow from the lungs to connect to the back wall of the left atrium. These veins are called the pulmonary veins, and they become the route for blood to pass from the lungs back to the heart to be pumped out to the body. In the normal child, two veins connect from the right lung and two from the left lung. In the condition known as *total anomalous pulmonary venous return* (TAPVR), these lung veins do not connect to the left atrium at all. Instead, they come together to form a common vein that attaches directly or indirectly to the right atrium. The condition is also known as *total anomalous pulmonary venous connection.*

The most common form of TAPVR **(A)** connects the lung veins to the superior vena cava, the blood vessel that brings oxygen-poor blue blood from the upper body back to the heart. Another form of TAPVR connects the lung veins to the coronary sinus, the pathway that carries blue blood from the heart muscle itself back to the right atrium. The common lung veins may also connect directly to the back of the right atrium.

The most unusual form of TAPVR **(B)** occurs when the common lung veins connect to the inferior vena cava, the blood vessel that brings blue blood from the lower body back to the heart. To reach the inferior vena cava, the lung veins must extend below the diaphragm, the division between the chest and abdomen. This type of defect, called an infradiaphragmatic TAPVR, may also include an obstruction between the common lung veins and the right atrium. The lungs quickly become congested and the baby will have respiratory failure.

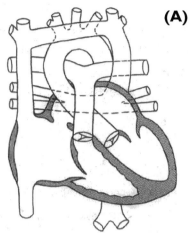

(A)

Total Anomalous Pulmonary Venous Connection to Left Vertical Vein (Supracardiac)

Atrial Septal Defect (Secundum)

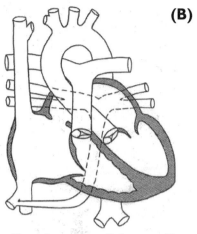

(B)

Total Anomalous Pulmonary Venous Connection to Ductus Venosus (Infradiaphragmatic)

Atrial Septal Defect

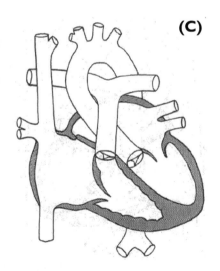

(C)

Partial Anomalous Pulmonary Venous Connection

(Right Pulmonary Veins to Junction of Superior Vena Cava & Right Atrium)

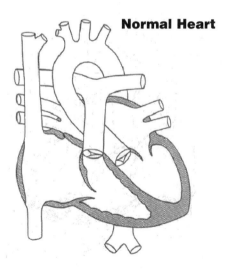

Normal Heart

Please refer to page 11 for a detailed illustration of the normal heart.

In all cases of TAPVR, a hole is present between the upper chambers of the heart, called an atrial septal defect. The hole is necessary for some blood to pass to the left side of the heart so it can be pumped out to the body. In a baby with TAPVR, the oxygen-poor blue blood returns to the right atrium, as normal, but then mixes with the pink blood coming from the lungs through one of the abnormal connections described above. Some of the mixed blood will follow the normal route to the lungs and some will cross through the atrial septal defect to get to the left side of the heart and be pumped out to the body.

The baby may develop signs of heart failure, such as fast breathing, poor feeding and failure to gain weight well. The baby may also have a heart murmur. Oxygen saturation in the blood will also be lower than normal.

TAPVR can only be repaired by surgery. The operation involves opening the back of the left atrium, sewing the common veins directly to the wall of the left atrium, and closing off the abnormal blood vessel to the right side of the heart. The atrial septal defect is also closed at this time.

A similar condition called a *partial anomalous pulmonary venous return (PAPVR)* **(C)** involves one or two pulmonary veins connecting abnormally instead of all four. Usually, an atrial septal defect is also present. Many times, the only symptom in the child is a heart murmur. PAPVR is repaired by creating a tunnel within the right atrium using tissue from the pericardium, the sac-like membrane around the heart. This tunnel is connected to the atrial septal defect, to allow oxygen-rich pink blood from the pulmonary veins to pass to the left atrium, as it would normally.

Transposition of the Great Arteries

In *transposition of the great arteries,* the aorta comes off the right ventricle and the pulmonary artery arises from the left ventricle **(A)**. The aorta will then take unoxygenated blood back to the body, before it can flow to the lungs for oxygen. The pulmonary artery takes blood from the left side of the heart back to the lungs. Infants born with transposition of the great arteries will be blue or "cyanotic" at birth or soon after birth, because unoxygenated blood is being delivered to the body.

Before birth, the normal fetus has a hole in the wall between the atria, the upper two chambers of the heart. This opening is called a patent foramen ovale, or PFO. There is also a vessel between the pulmonary artery and the aorta outside the heart called a patent ductus arteriosus, or PDA. If the structures remain open after the baby is born, blood will mix at these structures and some oxygenated blood will get to the body. However, these structures are not meant to stay open long after birth and will eventually close, allowing poorly oxygenated blood to get to the body. If the PFO is critically small, the cardiologist will do a Rashkind balloon septostomy. During this procedure, a catheter is inserted through the big vein in the baby's groin. It is threaded up into the heart and across the PFO. Then the tiny balloon at the end of the catheter is inflated and pulled back through the PFO to make it bigger. This allows mixing of the unoxygenated and oxygenated blood so that more oxygenated blood will get to the body. Because there is still mixing of blood, the baby will still be blue, but less blue than prior to the septostomy.

• Surgery

The surgery that is most commonly done to repair this defect is the arterial switch or Jatene operation. It is open-heart surgery and the heart is stopped during the surgery. The aorta is cut above the level of the coronary arteries. The pulmonary artery is cut at the same level. The coronary arteries are removed from the remaining base of the aorta and then reattached to the base of the pulmonary artery. Then the aorta is sewn to the base of the pulmonary artery and the pulmonary artery is sewn to the base of the aorta, essentially "switching" the circulation and preserving the coronary circulation. The aorta now comes off the left ventricle and can carry the oxygenated blood to the body. The pulmonary artery comes off the right ventricle, ready to carry the blood to the lungs for oxygen. During the surgery, the ASD that was created during the Rashkind balloon septostomy will also be closed by sewing a Gore-Tex patch over the hole.

Transposition of the Great Arteries With Ventricular Septal Defect (B)

Roughly 30-40% of patients with transposition of the great arteries (see above) also have ventricular septal defect, or VSD. This is a hole in the wall, or septum, between the two lower chambers of the heart, the ventricles. This hole will allow unoxygenated and oxygenated blood to mix so that some oxygen can get to the body.

• **Surgery**

The surgery that is most commonly done to repair this defect is the arterial switch or Jatene operation, described above, in addition to ventricular septal defect patch closure.

Transposition of the Great Arteries with Ventricular Septal Defect and Left Ventricular Outflow Obstruction (C)

About 30% of patients with transposition of the great arteries and ventricular septal defects also have an obstruction to the flow of blood out of the left ventricle, or subpulmonary stenosis. This may be caused by the wall, or septum, between the ventricles bowing or curving into the left ventricle, causing a blockage to the flow of blood out of that ventricle.

• **Surgery**

In patients who have transposition of the great arteries, a VSD, and severe subpulmonary stenosis, a Rastelli procedure is performed. A Rastelli procedure is a general term used for operations where a "conduit," or tube-like connection is placed from the right ventricle to the pulmonary artery, bypassing the blockage near the pulmonary valve. A tunnel is also created to direct the flow of blood from the left ventricle to the aorta, closing the VSD. This procedure is open-heart surgery and the heart is stopped during the surgery. It is usually done when the baby is close to one year of age. When successfully completed, the aorta now comes off the left ventricle and can carry the oxygenated blood to the body. The pulmonary artery comes off the right ventricle, ready to carry the blood to the lungs for oxygen. Unfortunately the right ventricular to pul-

(A)

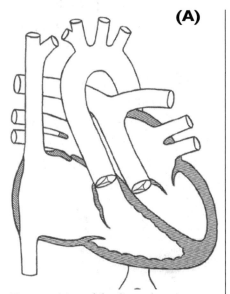

Transposition of the Great Arteries
Left Aortic Arch
Intact Ventricular Septum

(B)

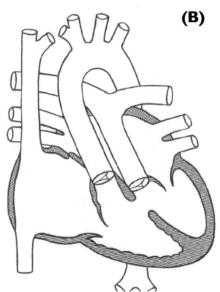

Transposition of the Great Arteries
Ventricular Septal Defect

(C)

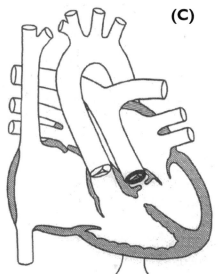

Transposition of the Great Arteries

Ventricular Septal Defect

Pulmonary Stenosis
  Valvular
  Discrete Subvalvular

Normal Heart

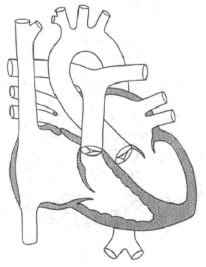

Please refer to page 11 for a detailed
illustration of the normal heart.

monary artery conduit does not grow with the child and will have to be replaced. Therefore, further procedures will have to be done to alleviate the right ventricle to pulmonary artery conduit narrowing over time.

Tricuspid Atresia

Normally, the tricuspid valve allows oxygen-poor blue blood to pass from the right atrium to the right ventricle, where it is pumped through the pulmonary artery to the lungs to pick up oxygen. In *tricuspid atresia* **(A)**, however, the tricuspid valve is not present. The only way for blue blood to get to the right ventricle is through a hole in the wall between the right and left atria. This hole, called an atrial septal defect, allows oxygen-poor blue blood to mix with oxygen-rich pink blood in the left side of the heart and travel to the left ventricle where it is pumped out the aorta and throughout the body. This mixing of the blood will create a slight bluish color in the child, called cyanosis.

Several other heart defects may also be present in the child with tricuspid atresia, including ventricular septal defect, pulmonary stenosis and transposition of the great arteries.

If the child also has ventricular septal defect, or a hole in the heart between the two ventricles, excessive blood will pass to the lungs instead of out to the body. This creates extra work for the heart and lungs, and may result in symptoms of congestive heart failure, such as fast breathing, poor feeding and failure to gain weight well.

Pulmonary stenosis, another problem commonly seen in children with tricuspid atresia, is a blockage in the artery that carries blood to the lungs. If the blockage is severe, insufficient blood travels to the lungs and the baby's oxygen levels may be inadequate.

The third problem often associated with tricuspid atresia is transposition of the great vessels in which the pulmonary artery and the aorta are connected to the wrong chambers of the heart **(B)**.

Regardless of the problems associated with tricuspid atresia, however, the baby will likely require the same ultimate surgical repair: a two-stage combination of

(A)

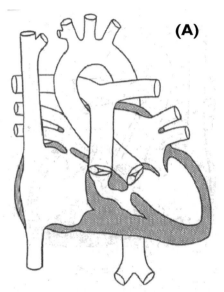

Tricuspid Valve Atresia
Ventricular Septal Defect (Restrictive)
Hypoplastic Right Ventricle
Small Atrial Septal Defect

(B)

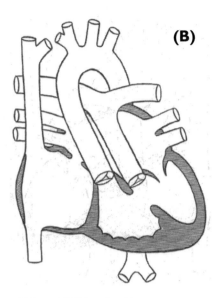

Tricuspid Valve Atresia
Transposition of the Great Arteries
Ventricular Septal Defect
Atrial Septal Defect
Small Right Ventricle

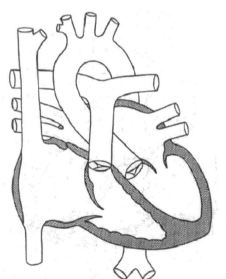

Normal Heart

*Please refer to page 11
for a detailed illustration
of the normal heart.*

the Glenn shunt and a Fontan procedure. If pulmonary blood flow is excessive, a preliminary operation, called a pulmonary band procedure, is required. If pulmonary blood flow is markedly reduced, a BT shunt may be needed.

Usually when the baby reaches six to twelve months of age, the Glenn shunt will be done to connect the superior vena cava directly to the pulmonary artery. The superior vena cava is the large vein that brings blue blood from the upper body to the heart. Most commonly, surgeons complete a bidirectional Glenn shunt, which allows blood to go to both the right and left lungs.

The Fontan procedure, usually done when the baby reaches 2-4 years of age, connects the inferior vena cava directly to the pulmonary artery. The inferior vena cava is the blood vessel that brings blue blood from the lower body to the heart. Because the inferior vena cava is not near the pulmonary artery, a tunnel must be created within the right atrium to make this connection, called a lateral tunnel Fontan.

In some children, a small hole, or fenestration, is left in the lateral tunnel Fontan conduit as a "pop-off" provision, in case high pressure develops in the connection between the inferior vena cava and the pulmonary artery. While on the heart-lung machine during surgery, the child's lungs tend to take on a little extra fluid and to become stiffer, which in turn causes lung pressure to be higher and creates more work to get blood into the pulmonary artery. The "pop-off" allows some blue blood to escape to the left side of the heart to maintain a lower pressure on the right side. A few months after surgery, the body tends to adjust to the Fontan repair, and the small hole, or fenestration, will either close on its own or can be closed surgically or via a cardiac catheterization device. No fenestration of the Fontan will be performed in patients whom the physicians do not believe will have fluid retention problems.

The Glenn shunt and Fontan procedures can be done at the same time in some patients, but doctors usually prefer to do the operations at least six to twelve months apart for the safety of the child.

Truncus Arteriosus

Truncus arteriosus means that there is one common vessel or trunk from the heart instead of a separate pulmonary artery and aorta. There is only one valve between the heart and this trunk. Normally, the pulmonary artery carries the pulmonary circulation, the blood that goes to the lungs, and the aorta carries the systemic circulation, the blood that goes throughout the rest of the body.

In truncus arteriosus, the trunk carries both the pulmonary and systemic circulation as well as the coronary circulation, which normally arises off the aorta. The trunk overrides both ventricles and there is always a ventricular septal defect (VSD), a hole in the wall between the lower two chambers of the heart. In truncus arteriosus, the oxygenated blood mixes with unoxygenated blood in the heart through the VSD. All the blood goes through the trunk and can either proceed through the trunk or go into the pulmonary artery and go to the lungs without ever carrying oxygen to the body. This explains why the baby can be blue, or "cyanotic," because some of the unoxygenated blood goes to the systemic circulation. There are four types of this congenital heart defect.

Type I

In truncus arteriosus type I **(A)**, which makes up more than 50% of the four types, the main pulmonary artery branches off the trunk, then further divides into the right pulmonary artery and the left pulmonary artery. The blood leaves the heart through the trunk and some of it will go into the pulmonary artery. Blood that does not go into the pulmonary artery will proceed through the trunk to the body and the coronary arteries. The blood that has entered the main pulmonary artery will then divide through the right pulmonary artery to the right lung and through the left pulmonary artery to the left lung.

Type II

In truncus arteriosus type II **(B)**, which makes up about 20% of this type of defect, there is no main pulmonary artery. The left and the right pulmonary arteries come off the back of the trunk, close to each other, but separately, each carrying blood to the lungs, the left pulmonary artery carrying blood to the left lung and the right pulmonary artery carrying blood to the right lung.

When blood leaves the heart through the trunk, some of it will proceed through these arteries to the lungs. The rest of the blood will go through the trunk to the systemic and the coronary circulations.

Type III

In truncus arteriosus type III (B), the pulmonary arteries come out of the sides of the trunk remote from each other. This defect accounts for about 10% of all truncus arteriosus. There is no main pulmonary artery. The left and the right pulmonary arteries come off the trunk separately, each carrying blood to the lungs, the left pulmonary artery carrying blood to the left lung and the right pulmonary artery carrying blood to the right lung. When blood leaves the heart through the trunk, some of it goes through these arteries to the lungs. The rest of the blood goes through the trunk to the systemic and the coronary circulation.

Type IV

Truncus arteriosus type IV (C) is also known as pseudotruncus, and can also be considered a form of pulmonary atresia with ventricular septal defect (VSD) with MAPCAs. The term is rarely used anymore.

• Surgery

Because excess blood can repeatedly go to the lungs, the lungs get "flooded." To restrict the blood from going to the lungs, a pulmonary artery banding can be performed early in life. Pulmonary artery banding is usually not open-heart surgery, and the heart does not need to be stopped. A "band," usually made of Gore-Tex, a material similar to rain gear, is placed around the pulmonary artery. This, in essence, kinks the pulmonary artery and restricts the blood from going to the lungs and forces it to the body. Pulmonary artery banding is a palliative procedure—a fix, not a cure. Complete repair is usually a modification of a Rastelli procedure. Generally, a Rastelli procedure connects the right ventricle to the pulmonary artery using a tube-like connection. This tube is usually a homograft, made from human cadaver tissue. During the Rastelli procedure, the ventricular septal defect is closed with a Gore-Tex patch so that the aorta arises solely from the LV.

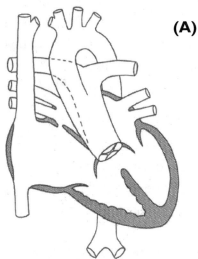

(A)

Truncus Arteriosus (Type I)

Ventricular Septal Defect

*Atrial Septal Defect
(vs. Patent Foramen Ovale)*

Left Aortic Arch

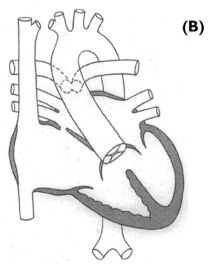

(B)

Truncus Arteriosus (Type II-III)

Ventricular Septal Defect

Atrial Septal Defect

Left Aortic Arch

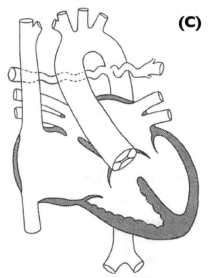

(C)

Truncus Arteriosus (Type IV)
Ventricular Septal Defect
Atrial Septal Defect
Left Aortic Arch
Separate Systemic Collaterals to each Lung

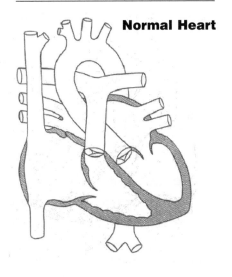

Normal Heart

*Please refer to page 11
for a detailed illustration
of the normal heart.*

Ventricular Septal Defect (VSD)

A *ventricular septal defect* (VSD) is a hole in the partition, or septum, between the two lower pumping chambers (ventricles) of the heart. This is the most common congenital heart defect. This hole allows blood to cross from the left ventricle, where the pressure is high, into the right ventricle, where the pressure is much lower. The larger the hole, the more blood will cross from the left to the right side.

Children with a VSD often will have a loud heart murmur after the first few weeks of life. Early in the newborn period, the pressure in the lungs and the right ventricle are higher than usual. This high pressure in the right ventricle prevents a lot of blood from crossing the VSD in the first days and weeks after the baby is born. The heart murmur at this time may be very soft, or absent, and the baby may not have any symptoms. When the lung and right ventricle pressure begin to fall to normal to low levels, more blood will cross the VSD and the heart murmur will get louder. The baby may begin to show signs of overcirculation, sometimes referred to as congestive heart failure. Signs of congestive heart failure include poor feeding, fast breathing even when the baby is sleeping, excessive sweating, poor weight gain, congestion and coughing. Severity of these symptoms and the age of onset depend upon the size of the hole—the larger the hole, the greater the severity of symptoms and the earlier they will appear. Many babies with a large VSD will have some symptoms of congestive heart failure by the time they are two months old.

Initial treatment of VSD often is with medication to help the heart and lungs deal with the increased workload. If treatment with medicine is successful at controlling congestive heart failure, your doctor may advise waiting for the VSD to close by itself. If the hole is small, no treatment may be needed. Medications may include digoxin, which helps the heart beat more strongly, and Lasix, which helps the baby's body get rid of water.

Additional medications, such as captopril, which helps the blood vessels in the body relax to decrease the amount of work the heart must pump against, may also be prescribed.

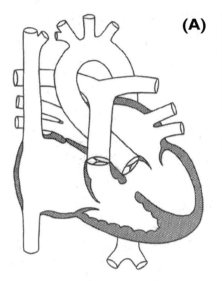

(A)

*Interventricular Septal Defect
(Perimembranous)*

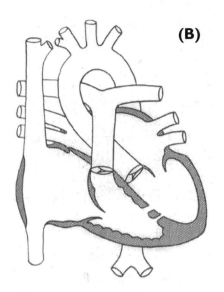

(B)

*Muscular Interventricular
Septal Defects*

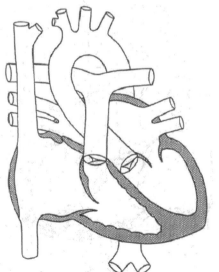

Normal Heart

*Please refer to page 11
for a detailed illustration
of the normal heart.*

In addition to medication, a child with VSD may be placed on a high calorie formula. Normally, formula and breast milk contain 20 calories per ounce. To help the baby gain weight, doctors may recommend mixing normal formula with less water or adding powdered formula to breast milk to increase the amount of calories per ounce.

• **Surgery will be recommended if:**

1. Congestive heart failure persists or the baby does not gain weight well, even on maximal medical treatment.

2. Persistent high pressure in the lungs due to the VSD is likely to cause permanent damage.

3. Other parts of the heart can potentially be affected by letting the hole remain open.

4. There is persistent cardiac enlargement over time.

Two forms of ventricular septal defect are common. Membranous VSD **(A)**, also known as peri-membranous defect, occurs when the hole in the septum does not contain muscle tissue. This defect is close to the heart valves, in particular the aortic and tricuspid valves, which may become involved with the VSD. The other form, muscular VSD **(B)**, occurs when holes in the muscle wall occur all over the septum. If these holes are large, they may require early surgical closure. Small muscular defects have a good chance of closing without surgery. If these holes are located in the RV outflow tract, known as conal or supracristal VSDs, they may require surgical closure even if they are small because of the possible danger to the nearby aortic valve.

Acquired Heart Conditions

Arrhythmia

The heart's rhythm must be carefully coordinated to pump blood efficiently throughout the body. To accomplish this coordination normally, the heart relies on an elaborate electrical system that stimulates the muscular walls of the atria and ventricles to contract and relax in sequence.

The heart's electrical system is composed of the sinus node, the AV (atrio-ventricular) node, the bundle branch conduction pathways, and most of the muscle cells of the atria and ventricles. Each heartbeat starts with an electrical impulse from the sinus node, which is the normal pacemaker of the body. The impulse then travels along the other parts of the electrical system to activate the atria and the ventricles, thereby completing a single heartbeat. Damage to any part of the heart's electrical system can result in an abnormally slow heart rate, called *bradycardia*, or an abnormally fast heart rate, called *tachycardia*.

Children can have serious heart rhythm problems before or immediately after birth, most often with heart rates that are too fast. Rhythm problems can be congenitally acquired, but may not become troublesome until much later. They can result from viral infections or can occur after heart surgery.

Bradycardia

Bradycardia, or slow heart rate, may be caused by an abnormally slow activity of the sinus node or conduction blockage somewhere within the electrical system, a condition called heart block. Heart block can occur as only a delay in conduction of the impulses from the atria to the ventricles, called first degree block, or intermittently blocked impulses, called second degree block, or completely blocked impulses, called third degree block. Some patients may be born with heart block (congenital block). Other patients may develop heart block because of a medication, abnormal blood chemistries, inflammation, or after surgery. Bradycardia may cause symptoms such as fatigue, poor exercise tolerance, dizziness, and syncope (loss of consciousness). Rarely, profound bradycardia may lead to death.

Pacemakers

Bradycardia and its associated symptoms may be improved or prevented with insertion of a permanent pacemaker. This mechanical device provides an electrical trigger for a heart beat when and where it is needed.

A typical pacemaker consists of one or two pacing leads that connect to a pulse generator, which contains a battery and circuitry, including a computer chip. Some pacemakers have special sensors that measure how active a patient is, allowing for more normal range of heart rates (e.g., slower rate at rest and faster rate with exercise).

Patients who receive a pacemaker with only one pacing lead have a single chamber pacemaker; those with two leads have a dual chamber pacemaker. Epicardial pacing leads are implanted on the outer surface of the heart and the pulse generator is placed in the abdominal region. This is often the approach of choice for infants and small children. In contrast, transvenous, or endocardial, pacing leads are commonly used in adults and older children. These leads are passed through one of the upper veins leading into the heart using X-ray guidance and the pulse generator is placed in the shoulder region.

Pacemakers are usually implanted under general anesthesia, and the patient remains in the hospital for one to several days. Patients are typically seen in the outpatient clinic soon after hospital discharge, and then every 6 to 12 months thereafter. In addition to these visits, periodic telephone follow-up is accomplished using a special device called a transmitter. In general, a patient with a pacemaker can participate in most routine physical activities and have few restrictions to daily living.

Tachycardia

Tachycardia, or fast heart rate, may result from abnormal electrical activity from electrical "short circuits" or abnormal activity of a small group of heart cells. This may occur in the absence of obvious heart disease, or may be associated with heart disease such as those who have undergone cardiac surgery. Symptoms of tachycardia include palpitations, dizziness, shortness of breath, and syncope (fainting). Serious forms of tachycardia can lead to sudden death. Depending upon clinical circumstances, tachycardia can be treated with medications, electrical therapy, radio-frequency ablation using catheters, or heart surgery.

Medications

A variety of medications are used to treat patients with tachycardia. No medicine can eliminate or permanently change the tissues of the heart causing the tachycardia, but many medicines may effectively stop tachycardia or prevent its recurrence. Although "antiarrhythmic" medications are generally well tolerated, most can cause side effects. Medications most commonly used in pediatric arrhythmia management include:

Adenosine is a medicine commonly used in the emergency room to abruptly stop tachycardia due to supraventricular tachycardia. Adenosine can only be given using an IV, and is usually very effective. Adenosine lasts only 10 seconds in the bloodstream, so it cannot be used as a long-term medicine to prevent recurrent tachycardia.

Digoxin is one of the most widely prescribed medications in children with heart disease. It is most often used to increase the squeezing strength (contractile force) of each heartbeat. Digoxin also slows down the heart rate during some types of tachycardia by increasing the activity of the parasympathetic nervous system. However, digoxin is not a powerful way to treat arrhythmias and may be combined with other antiarrhythmic medications. Although generally well tolerated, possible side effects include nausea, vomiting, visual changes, and tiredness, especially if too much medicine is ingested. Some other medications alter the way digoxin is absorbed in the body, so dosage may need to be adjusted.

Beta blockers, such as propanolol (Inderal), atenolol (Tenormin), and metoprolol (Lopressor) are common medicines used to prevent tachycardia. These drugs block the sympathetic nervous system and slow activity in the "beta receptors" in the heart, causing abnormal heart rate to slow down. The side effects of beta blockers include bradycardia, hypotension, fatigue, and mood swings. Patients with asthma may have problems with breathing. Small children must eat or drink regularly, as beta blockers may affect blood sugar levels. This is especially important in young children when they are sick and have a poor appetite.

Amiodarone (Cordarone) and **sotalol** (Betapace) are medicines that are used when others have failed to treat tachycardia. These drugs have many actions, including the blockage of potassium, calcium channels and beta receptors in the heart. It is recommended that these medications be initiated in the hospital where the heart rhythm can be continuously monitored because of the potential for serious side effects, most notably serious arrhythmias. The medications may also require periodic blood tests to assess effects on other organs of the body. Some side effects seen with these medications are bradycardia, heart block, arrhythmias, skin sensitivity to the sun, vision disturbances, thyroid disorders, changes in lung function, liver or blood changes.

Electrical Therapy
When tachycardia is dangerous and cannot be controlled by medication, immediate electrical therapy may be needed to terminate the fast rhythm. Electrical therapy involves delivering electrical impulses directly to the atrial or ventricular tissue to stop tachycardia. These impulses can be delivered in several ways:

- A transesophageal lead or wire can be inserted through the nose and placed in the esophagus, which lies immediately behind the heart. This lead can be used to deliver electrical impulses to the heart, often stopping tachycardia. Mild sedation is often necessary to help the patient relax and decrease discomfort during this form of treatment. Occasionally, a transesophageal pacing study is used to determine which types of tachycardia a patient may have, or to evaluate the effectiveness of medication in preventing future episodes of tachycardia.

- Implantable antitachycardia devices are similar to pacemakers, but can also automatically deliver electrical therapy to stop tachycardia abruptly. These devices constantly monitor the patient's heart rhythm, and terminate tachycardia soon after it begins. Antitachycardia devices can decrease the need for medications and reduce emergency room visits for episodes of tachycardia. Most patients do not feel the therapies delivered by antitachycardia pacemakers. These devices may also prevent the heart from going too slow.

- Implantable cardioverter-defibrillators (ICDs) are another type of automatic device most commonly used to treat very dangerous forms of tachycardia, such as ventricular tachycardia. Most ICDs are implanted using the transvenous approach. Cardiac rhythms are constantly monitored and when a ventricular tachycardia occurs, the device can deliver a shock to the heart muscle. Most patients feel some discomfort during the therapy, but sudden death may occur without the shock. Patients with ICDs are followed in the outpatient clinic every 3 to 4 months. Patients generally have few restrictions to daily living, and can participate in many less strenuous physical activities, except as limited by underlying heart disease.

RF Catheter Ablation

This procedure is used to eliminate the source of the problem in some types of tachycardia. The cardiologist performs this procedure in the cardiac catheterization lab, usually with the patient under general anesthesia. Catheters or wires are placed into the patient's heart by way of large veins in the legs and neck. The cardiologist then "maps" the heart's electrical system to locate the electrical short-circuit or over-active cells. Once found, this small amount of abnormal tissue can be ablated, or destroyed, by direct heating of the tip of a special catheter using radio-frequency current. Preventing the tissue area from causing future episodes of tachycardia eliminates the need for medicines or other treatments.

Cardiomyopathy

Cardiomyopathy is a disease of the heart muscle, often without an identifiable cause. It can be associated with skeletal muscle diseases, such as Friedreich's ataxia, muscular dystrophy, or glycogen storage disease, or with viral infections. It is usually chronic and can result in dilated cardiomyopathy, which is a weakened heart muscle, or restrictive cardiomyopathy, which is a stiff heart muscle. Hypertrophic cardiomyopathy (also known as idiopathic hypertrophic subaortic stenosis, or IHSS, or as asymmetric septal hypertrophy or ASH) can occur in families. With these conditions, the left ventricular muscle, especially the septal wall separating the right and the left ventricles, becomes extremely thickened and can obstruct the exit of blood into the aorta. The thickened muscle is prone to heart rhythm irregularities.

Congestive Heart Failure

The heart has two pumping systems—the right side, which pumps blood to the lungs, and the left side, which pumps blood to the body. Congestive heart failure develops when the pumping action of the heart deteriorates to the point that the heart is unable to pump enough blood to meet the body's needs. This may occur as a result of an excessive workload on the heart muscle.

One way the heart responds to an excessive workload is by beating faster to meet the body's demand for blood and oxygen. While this may have a short-term benefit, over time the heart can become enlarged, causing the muscle walls of the heart to grow weak and inefficient. This can reduce blood volume in the body, which causes the body's arteries to constrict, forcing the heart to work even harder to pump blood. Eventually, blood will back up into the lungs and in other areas of the body, such as the liver and extremities. When blood backs up, it isn't delivered properly throughout the body, which places further demand on the heart to beat faster, which leads to further deterioration.

Congestive Heart Failure in Children

Congenital heart defects are the most common cause for heart failure in infancy and childhood. These include: hypoplastic left heart syndrome, coarctation of the aorta, ventricular septal defects, patent ductus arteriosus, atrioventricular canal, total anomalous pulmonary venous connections, transposition of the great arteries and truncus arteriosus. Primary myocardial diseases, such as myocarditis or cardiomyopathies, may evoke heart failure at any time. In addition, heart failure may occur after open-heart repair of congenital heart defects.

Other heart conditions that are acquired may lead to congestive heart failure after one year of age. These include: cardiomyopathies, rheumatic heart disease and severe cardiac dysrhythmias. High blood pressure from any cause may also lead to cardiac failure due to prolonged resistance in the blood vessels.

Signs and Symptoms

Signs of heart failure will differ depending on the patient's age. In infants, a fast heart rate (greater than 160 beats per minute), difficulty breathing and/or sweating during feeding can be the first signs of heart failure. As the disease progresses, the infant may not grow. When severe, congestive heart failure causes the infant to have fast and labored breathing, sometimes with grunting.

In older children and adults, heart failure is recognized by limitations in physical activity. In mild failure, the patient is comfortable at rest, but moderate physical activity causes fatigue, shortness of breath and occasionally palpitations and chest pain. As symptoms progress, minimal physical activity causes fatigue and other symptoms. Finally, in its most severe stage, heart failure causes the patient to be unable to carry on daily activities without symptoms or discomfort, and shortness of breath or chest pain may occur even at rest.

Treatment

The goal of treatment is to reduce the workload of the heart by controlling excess salt and water, thereby improving the heart's ability to pump. Medications also can be very effective in working toward that goal. These medications include: ACE inhibitors, such as captopril, to open the arteries and veins so more blood can reach the body's tissues; diuretics, such as Lasix, to act on the kidneys to rid the body of extra salt and water, reducing the accumulation of fluid in the lungs to lower blood pressure and improve the efficiency of blood circulation; and digoxin, which helps treat congestive heart failure by increasing the strength of the heart's contractions.

New research studies are looking at medications to block the sympathetic activity of the heart, that part of the nervous system that causes an increase in heart rate and blood pressure. Beta blockers, such as carvedilol, block the activity of the sympathetic nervous system and may be effective in slowing the progression of congestive heart failure.

Endocarditis

Endocarditis is a disease of the inner lining of the heart. It can be associated with generalized systemic inflammatory diseases, such as lupus erythematosus or Liebman-Sachs, and results in thickened and distorted heart valves. Rheumatic fever may cause similar valve damage. Infectious endocarditis is caused by bacterial bloodstream infections. It can develop rapidly, an acute condition, or slowly, a sub-acute condition. Children with certain congenital or acquired heart disease are sensitive to this infection. (*For more information on bacterial endocarditis, see Chapter Nine.*)

Pericarditis

Pericarditis is an inflammatory disease of the outer lining of the heart, which normally has a sack-like double layer with a small amount of fluid inside for lubrication. When inflamed, the amount of fluid increases and can compress the heart to the point of malfunction. When infected, pus can accumulate in the pericardial sac, known as purulent pericarditis. Occasionally, there is not enough fluid between the layers and the smooth inner surfaces become rough, causing pain with each heartbeat, a condition known as fibrinous pericarditis.

Rheumatic Heart Disease

Rheumatic heart disease is caused by **Streptococcus bacterium,** usually associated with a sore throat, commonly known as "strep throat." It starts as rheumatic fever and can involve the joints, the kidney, and the heart. It can affect the heart muscle, a condition known as myocarditis; the mitral and/or aortic valves, a condition called valvulitis; or the outer membrane of the heart, a condition known as pericarditis. When the acute insult is over, it can leave behind leaky regurgitant valves. These conditions can be prevented by early treatment of streptococcal throat infections. Once a child develops heart disease from streptococcal infection, he or she must remain on antibiotics for life to prevent recurrence that can further damage the heart valves.

Viral Myocarditis

Viral myocarditis can be caused by a variety of viruses. Occasionally, it may damage the heart muscle permanently, a condition known as cardiomyopathy.

Diagnostic Tests

There are several diagnostic tests that may be used to identify a heart problem or check the status of a previous surgical procedure. Among the more common tests are:

Cardiac Catheterization

Diagnostic Catheterization

In this invasive procedure, a hollow tube or catheter is inserted into a vein in the arm or leg and then moved up into the heart. A contrast dye is injected and fluoroscopic pictures are taken of the heart chambers, blood vessels and heart valves. The pressures and oxygen content of the different heart chambers can also be measured. Usually a few weeks before the procedure, the physician will order pre-operative testing (such as a chest X-ray, EKG, echocardiogram and/or blood work). Your child will come to the hospital on the morning of the procedure and will receive sedation. Recovery will require several hours after the procedure. During this time, the nurses will monitor blood pressure, pulse, the insertion site for signs of bleeding, and pulse oximetry, a measurement of the amount of oxygen in the blood.

Interventional Catheterization

These procedures are similar to diagnostic catheterization, except the goal is placement of the catheter to treat an underlying condition.

Balloon Angioplasty

This procedure is used to correct a narrow blood vessel by inserting a balloon-tipped catheter and inflating the balloon at the point of narrowing to stretch the blood vessel.

Balloon Valvuloplasty

Similar to balloon angioplasty, this procedure is used to correct a narrow valve by inserting a balloon-tipped catheter and inflating the balloon at the point of narrowing to stretch the valve.

Arrhythmia Ablation

This procedure uses specially designed catheters that are inserted into heart chambers to locate and then destroy, or ablate, the source or sources of heart rate irregularity.

Catheter Device Techniques

This procedure uses specially designed catheters to guide clotting materials or devices, such as coils, to close or occlude abnormal vessels or certain holes between heart chambers.

• Stents

Stents are placed in narrowed blood vessels around the heart, such as the pulmonary arteries. The stent is a small wire mesh tube, usually made out of stainless steel.

The stent is usually placed during a cardiac catheterization. The collapsed stent is placed over a tiny balloon near the end of a catheter. The catheter is advanced through the groin and then the balloon is positioned in the narrowed vessel. X-ray is used to help see the correct position of the stent. The balloon is then inflated and the stent expands, pushing the narrowed vessel open. The balloon is then deflated, and the catheter removed, leaving the stent in place. Patients need to take aspirin or other blood thinners for a period of time after the stent placement. This helps prevent blood from clotting around the stent until the body's own cells grow over the stent. Additionally, stents can be expanded or made larger, for example, as a child's vessels grow larger. This is done by reinserting a larger-ballooned catheter in the cardiac catheterization laboratory, and inflating the balloon, further expanding the stent in place.

• Septal Closure Devices

Holes in the septum (wall) of heart (ASDs, VSDs, or PFOs) can also be closed in the cardiac catheterization laboratory, using a septal closure device. This can be done instead of surgery, if the location, size and borders of the hole are appropriate. Those characteristics also determine which of several FDA approved devices may be appropriate to close the hole.

Devices are threaded up through a catheter that enters the patient through a blood vessel in the groin. The catheter is advanced across the hole and part of the device is pushed out into the chamber on the left side of the heart. The catheter is then pulled back to the right side of the heart, and the remainder of the device is pushed out, sandwiching the wall with the hole between the two sides of the device.

Devices are made of thin metal, some connected with fabric. The device closes the hole by covering both the left and right side of the septum. The device serves as a bridge, allowing the patients own cells to grow across it, completely sealing it. Patients need to take aspirin or other blood thinner for a period of time after device placement. This helps blood from clotting on the device until the body's own cells grow over the device.

Valve Replacement via Cardiac Catheterization
Valve replacement via cardiac catheterization can be performed with very low morbidity and mortality. At the present time, the patient must be fully grown for the procedure to be done, and certain clinical criteria must be met. The valve is threaded through the catheter like other devices. The diseased valve that is to be replaced may be stented open and the "catheter valve" is placed adjacent to this area. As of now, only pulmonary valve replacement via cardiac catheterization has been approved.

Chest X-ray
The chest X-ray is a noninvasive test that provides radiological pictures of the structures in the chest, such as the heart, lungs, ribs, and sternum, or breast bone. It also provides information as to the size and position of the heart. A chest X-ray is useful in the diagnosis of pneumonia, tumors, collapsed lung, congestive heart failure and/or rib fractures. In addition, it is used to check placement of tubes and catheters in the chest, such as central lines, chest tubes, or nasogastric tubes threaded through the nasal passage to reach the stomach.

The level of radiation exposure from a chest X-ray is minimal. However, with repeated X-rays, it is advisable to cover genital areas with an X-ray-proof shield.

Computerized Axial Tomography (CT Scan)

The CT scan, or CAT scan, is a computerized x-ray providing cross-sectional pictures of the chest, which show in great detail the internal structures and any abnormalities. Some CT scans may require contrast dye administered either by mouth or through an intravenous line. Because it is necessary for the patient to remain very still during the test, younger patients may require sedation.

Echocardiogram

An echocardiogram is a noninvasive test using ultrasound technology to produce a picture from the sound waves that reflect from the tissue or organ being examined. A transducer, which transforms input energy of one form into output energy of another form, is placed over the chest. The machine then produces high frequency sound waves, which bounce off the heart structures and are sent back through the transducer to be plotted onto a graphic recording. This test is useful in evaluating the structure and function of the heart and valves.

There are two types of echocardiograms: transthoracic, through the chest wall from the front; and transesophageal, through the feeding tube or esophagus, which shows the heart from the rear view.

Electrocardiogram (ECG/EKG)

The ECG (EKG) is a noninvasive test in which electrodes are placed on the arms, legs, and chest. A graphic tracing of the electrical activity of the heart is produced and can assist in detecting abnormalities in the rhythm and structure of the heart.

Electrophysiology Studies (EP Studies)

An EP study is an invasive measure of the heart's electrical activity. A hollow catheter is placed into the right atrium of the heart then electrical stimuli are delivered through the catheter, while EKGs and computers monitor the cardiac electrical response. This procedure is helpful in the diagnosis of difficult dysrrhythmias and conduction disturbances. The procedure is usually done in the cardiac catheterization lab.

Holter Monitor

The Holter Monitor is a 24-, 48-, or 72-hour continuous monitor of a patient's ECG. A logbook is kept of the different activities and times at which they take place so that they may be later correlated with the ECG tracing.

Magnetic Resonance Imaging (MRI)

This is a noninvasive test using non-X-ray magnetic waves to form cross-sectional plain pictures similar to those of a CT scan. This test may require administration of a contrast dye and/or sedation. An MRI test should not be done for those patients with pacemakers, mechanical prosthetic valves or other implanted medical devices.

Prebirth Testing

There are two types of prebirth testing. A level II ultrasound is similar to a regular pregnancy ultrasound, but with much more detailed imaging of the entire fetus. The other, a fetal echocardiogram, is a noninvasive transabdominal ultrasound test of the fetal heart that can be done, usually after 14 weeks of pregnancy when the baby's heart is large enough to get a clear picture.

Stress Testing

The stress test is used to evaluate the heart's response to physical stress. It reveals the heart muscle's response to increased oxygen demands and also the blood flow to the heart tissue. The patient's heart rate, electrical activity, blood pressure, and respiratory rate are all monitored during the test and EKG tracings are produced before, during, and after the procedure.

Stress testing can be done with physical exercise on a treadmill or a stationary bike or can be done by administering medications to induce a stress response on the heart.

Stress tests may be done in conjunction with echocardiography or other X-ray examinations of the heart.

Equipment

Great strides have been made in the quality of heart treatment available to-day, thanks in large part to advances in technology. Some of the equipment used to treat heart patients includes:

Chest Tube

These small tubes are placed into the space between the chest wall and the lung, called the pleural space. These are placed after heart surgery to prevent accumulation of body fluids. The chest tube collection chamber will accumulate drainage, which should typically diminish in amount each day.

Central IV Lines

An IV or intravenous line may be placed in a vein that leads to the right atrium of the heart. Its purpose is to deliver intravenous fluids, nutrients and/or medications. It may also be used to monitor central heart pressures.

An arterial line is a catheter placed into an artery, one of the vessels that pulsate, to measure blood pressure and oxygen levels.

Defibrillator System
(Implantable Cardioverter Defibrillator and Leads)

When the electrical activity in the heart is too rapid and chaotic to allow the heart to effectively pump blood to the body, an implantable cardioverter defibrillator (ICD) may be implanted to send a burst of strong electricity ("shock") to reset the electrical signals in the heart to beat in a consistent, regular manner. The defibrillator can also function like a pacemaker when the heart is beating too slowly or irregularly. Like a pacemaker, a defibrillator contains a battery and mini-computer, along with other electrical components to create enough energy to shock the heart. Leads (insulated wires) transmit information between the heart and the ICD, sensing the activity in the heart muscle and carrying electrical signals to the heart from the ICD.

Defibrillators typically last from 4-6 years, depending on use. Medical person-nel should check defibrillator and lead function periodically to ensure optimal treatment. A physician should be consulted prior to engaging in sport activity.

Endotracheal Tube (ET Tube)

This tube is inserted, usually through the mouth, into the windpipe, or trachea, to provide an airway. At the same time, the ET Tube can prevent intake of foreign material into the lungs. In adults, there is a cuff that is inflated to help hold this tube in place. It is also taped in place over the patient's mouth and nose.

Foley Catheter

A Foley catheter is a tube placed into the bladder to drain out urine. The tube is held in place by a small balloon, which is inflated in the bladder after insertion. Often after surgery, a patient's IV and oral intake as well as urinary output will be monitored closely.

Heart-Lung Bypass Machine

This machine is used during open-heart surgery to oxygenate and pump the blood through the body while the heart is temporarily stopped for surgical repair.

Heart Monitoring Equipment

Before, during, and after surgery, the patient will be monitored with equipment at the bedside. This equipment usually records heart rhythm, heart rate, respiratory rate, pulse oximetry (the measure of oxygen in the blood) and any central line pressure readings.

Nasogastric Tube (NG Tube)

This tube is placed through the nose into the stomach and is used to either keep the stomach empty by pumping out gastric contents or to convey food into the stomach.

NIRS Monitor

This small sensor device is placed across the forehead and lower back and measures oxygen delivery to the brain and abdominal organs and tissues.

Oxygen

Oxygen is a colorless, odorless and tasteless gas required for breathing. It can be delivered by room air, or through a tube called a nasal cannula, through a mask or a tent, or through the ET tube. The blood then carries oxygen to the different tissues in the body. Because oxygen provides support for combustion, it should never be used in the presence of a lighted cigarette or open flame, or where there is the possibility of an electrical spark.

Pacemaker System
(Implantable Pulse Generator and Leads)

When the heart beats too slowly or irregularly, a pacemaker may be implanted under the skin to improve and monitor the heart function. A pacemaker is a small, thin electronic device containing a battery and mini-computer that senses and responds to the electrical activity in the heart. When the heart does not generate consistent electrical activity on its own, the pacemaker artificially creates the electrical activity that will cause the heart to beat. A lead is an insulated wire that carries these impulses from the pacemaker to the heart and in reverse, carries information on the electrical activity in the heart to the pacemaker. Pacemakers typically last from 6-10 years, depending on use. Medical personnel should check pacemaker and lead function periodically to ensure optimal treatment. A physician should be consulted prior to engaging in sport activity.

Pulse Oximeter

This is a noninvasive sensor that is clipped to a patient's finger, ear, or toe to monitor blood oxygen levels.

Suction Procedure

A catheter is inserted into the ET (endotracheal) tube, mouth or nose and a vacuum is activated to clear the airway of any secretions or foreign bodies. Often sterile water or saline (salt solution) is used to liquefy thick secretions before suctioning.

Temporary Pacemaker

Often after open-heart surgery, it is necessary to use an external temporary pacemaker until any heart swelling resolves and the heart's own pace-making mechanism is restored. The temporary pacemaker is a small box, which is attached by wires to the patient's chest.

Ventilator/Respirator

This mechanical device ventilates the patient by providing air to and from the lungs. It allows for administration of oxygen and removal of carbon dioxide from the body. The machine is connected to the ET tube to assist with breathing.

Ventricular Assist Devices
Berlin Heart

The Berlin heart is a ventricular assist device. It works by helping the right ventricle of the heart pump blood to lungs and the left ventricle pump blood to the body. The Berlin heart comes in various sizes for a range of patients, including newborn babies. Most of the device is extracorporeal (outside the body); only the tubes are implanted in the heart. They emerge from small openings in the skin to enter the pump, a small round chamber. The system is run by a laptop computer. The Berlin heart is intended to be used as a bridge to recovery or as a bridge to transplant.

ECMO

ECMO, or extracorporeal membrane oxygenation, is a mechanical means of oxygenating and pumping the blood outside the body. This is done to rest the heart or lungs, or both, while they recover from surgery or as a bridge to surgery or heart transplantation. The surgeons will place the tubes inside the heart or in the blood vessels of the neck or groin to connect to the ECMO machine. ECMO specialists will be in charge of the machine constantly and work together with the bedside nurse in managing the circuit.

Surgical Procedures

Surgical Procedures For Treatment of Congenital and Acquired Heart Defects

Cardiovascular surgical procedures or operations may have one of several goals. *Anatomically corrective* procedures are required to make heart structures normal. *Physiologically corrective* procedures are required to separate and/or redirect the blue and pink blood circulations. These corrective procedures range from the relatively simple, such as closing or patching a hole or tying off a vessel, to the complex, such as switching vessels or rerouting blood streams. Most corrective operations require the use of a heart-lung machine, a cardio-pulmonary bypass pump. Some corrective surgical procedures provide complete correction of the normal physiology of the heart. Some corrective procedures provide an altered type of physiology of the heart and provide permanent palliation, such as the Fontan procedure.

Palliative procedures are required to improve, but not correct, an abnormal heart function. Palliative operations are performed to improve the heart function, usually in children too young for corrective surgery. The aim is to lessen cyanosis, to control heart failure, or to prepare the circulation for later repair.

Few heart operations are truly corrective; usually some lifetime follow up is required. Most surgeries can restore the heart and vessels to near normal performance and extend the life span.

Cardiovascular operations require the chest to be opened under general anesthesia. The approach is either through the midline of the chest, called a median sternotomy, or from either side of the chest, called a lateral thoracotomy. Minimally invasive heart surgery using small incisions is gaining popularity and doctors are hopeful that endoscopic surgery will soon be available for some cardiac defects. Endoscopic surgery uses a viewing tube to examine and treat internal structures without opening the body surgically. Prior to the surgery, you will be given chlorhexidine wipes, a topical antimicrobial agent used to help protect against surgical site infections, used by wiping on the skin the night before and day of surgery.

Some of the better-known heart operations are described below for quick reference. (See *Chapter Three for the currently recommended surgical procedure appropriate to a specific defect.*)

Arterial Switch

The arterial switch is the preferred anatomically corrective operation for both simple and complex forms of d-transposition of the great arteries because it restores the structure and the function of the heart to normal. The aorta and pulmonary artery are severed from their transposed origins and reconnected in such a way that they receive the correct blood from the correct ventricle. That is, after repair, the LV directs blood to the aorta and the RV sends blood to the LV. The arterial switch requires a separate transfer of the coronary arteries from the originally right-sided aortic stump to the new left-sided aortic root, the former pulmonary trunk.

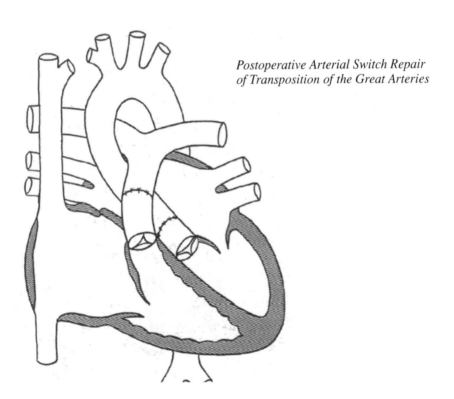

Postoperative Arterial Switch Repair of Transposition of the Great Arteries

The Blalock-Hanlon Procedure
(Creation of an Atrial Septal Defect)

This is a closed-heart operation aimed at improving the bluish cyanosis color in certain conditions such as transposition or tricuspid atresia. While complete separation of blue and pink circulations is normally desirable, in transposition and several other anomalies, the two circulations must mix within the heart for the child to do well. A hole in the atrial septum is an efficient way to accomplish such mixing. Eventually, anatomic or physiologic repair will follow.

The Blalock-Taussig or BT Shunt

Shunts are surgical connections, or anastomoses, between two arteries or between a vein and an artery. The Blalock-Taussig shunt connects a branch of the aorta, usually the subclavian artery, to the pulmonary artery directly or by using a plastic tube to increase the pulmonary blood flow.

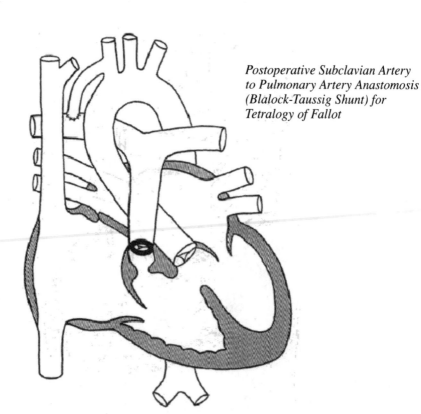

Postoperative Subclavian Artery to Pulmonary Artery Anastomosis (Blalock-Taussig Shunt) for Tetralogy of Fallot

Closure of Septal Defects

Smaller atrial and ventricular septal defects can be closed with sutures or stitches. Larger defects require the use of a plastic patch. Occasionally, in complex defects, the patch is used not only to close the hole between the ventricles but also to channel left ventricular blood through the right ventricle into the aorta through an intracardiac tunnel.

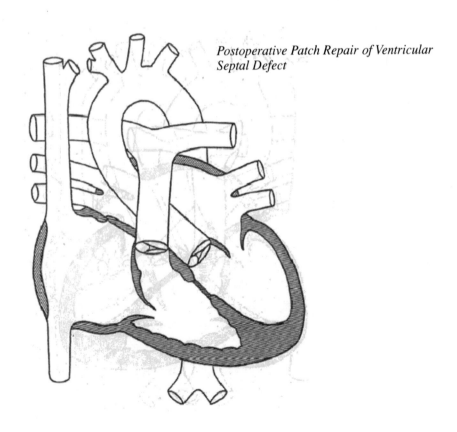

Postoperative Patch Repair of Ventricular Septal Defect

Correction of Narrow Valves

The four valves in the heart can be narrow (stenosed) or regurgitant (leaky), or both. They can be either repaired or replaced, depending on the nature of the problem. The most common aortic and pulmonic stenosis is caused by congenital fusion of one or more moving valve leaflets. Repair is done using cardiopulmonary bypass and by cutting the fused leaflets apart. Occasionally, however, the seat of the valve, the annulus, is small, a condition called hypoplastic. Enlargement of the pulmonic annulus is accomplished by cutting it and placing a trans-annular patch across it. The resulting valve leak is usually well tolerated for a decade or more. A small aortic annulus cannot be enlarged without valve replacement because it would cause excessive regurgitation, or leaking. A regurgitant aortic valve can sometimes be repaired by tightening the loose leaflets in a procedure called a valvuloplasty). Narrow mitral or tricuspid valves can rarely be enlarged and usually need to be replaced. Regurgitant mitral or tricuspid valves can frequently be repaired by valvuloplasty.

Valves can be replaced by biological or prosthetic material. Biological valves are either homograft, taken from a human cadaver donor, or porcine, taken from a pig. There is a variety of prosthetic valves available. Many issues need to be considered when choosing the most suitable valve. Mechanical prosthetic valves will require a lifetime of clot-preventing medication, such as Coumadin or aspirin, and may not be ideal for females desiring to become pregnant. At this writing, an ideal valve has not yet been designed and most prosthetic valves will eventually need replacement.

Damus-Kaye-Stansel Operation

This procedure usually complements other corrective procedures. It was originally developed along with the Rastelli procedure for correcting transposed great arteries with a VSD without switching them. It is now frequently employed as part of the Fontan operation in one-ventricle repairs to overcome any obstruction to the aortic blood flow. It consists of connecting the pulmonary trunk and the ascending aorta, and detaching the pulmonary artery branches. The pulmonary artery branches are supplied temporarily by an artificial shunt from the aortic branches. The aorta thus receives flow through both pulmonic and aortic valves.

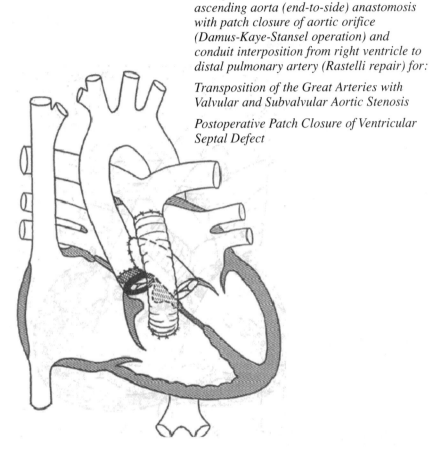

Postoperative main pulmonary artery to ascending aorta (end-to-side) anastomosis with patch closure of aortic orifice (Damus-Kaye-Stansel operation) and conduit interposition from right ventricle to distal pulmonary artery (Rastelli repair) for:

Transposition of the Great Arteries with Valvular and Subvalvular Aortic Stenosis

Postoperative Patch Closure of Ventricular Septal Defect

Double Switch Operation

This is an extensive surgical procedure combining the features of the arterial switch procedure and the Mustard procedure (venous switch). It is utilized for patients with ventricular inversion or congenitally corrected transposition of the great arteries. This procedure routes the pulmonary venous blood to the left atrium and then the aorta, and routes the systemic venous blood to the right ventricle and then the pulmonary artery. This procedure accomplishes the re-institution of the left ventricle as the systemic pump.

Fontan Operations

Many versions of this physiologically corrective procedure exist and they continue being updated. The Fontan operation is reserved for complex heart abnormalities that cannot undergo two-ventricle repair. Such hearts are grouped together as univentricular, meaning that there is only one functional ventricle, which must be left to propel the pink blood to the body. The blue and pink circulations are surgically separated by atrial partition and the blue side—the IVC, inferior vena cava and SVC, superior vena cava—is connected directly to the pulmonary artery without any valves. There is no pump for the blue blood, but the circulation is nevertheless effective as long as the pressure in the lungs are low. The operation eliminates the bluish cyanosis and allows for reasonable physical activities.

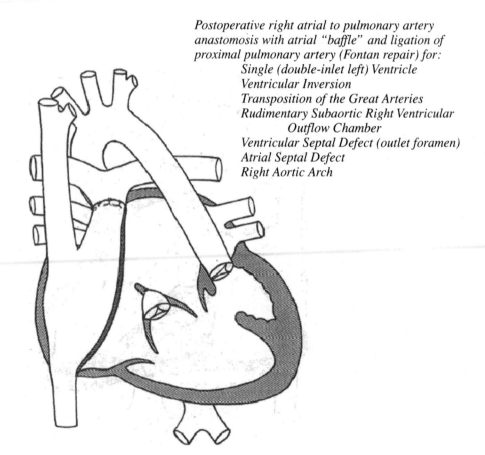

Postoperative right atrial to pulmonary artery anastomosis with atrial "baffle" and ligation of proximal pulmonary artery (Fontan repair) for:
  Single (double-inlet left) Ventricle
  Ventricular Inversion
  Transposition of the Great Arteries
  Rudimentary Subaortic Right Ventricular
      Outflow Chamber
  Ventricular Septal Defect (outlet foramen)
  Atrial Septal Defect
  Right Aortic Arch

Glenn Shunt

This closed surgical procedure connects the superior vena cava (SVC) directly to the pulmonary artery. In the classic Glenn shunt, the SVC was connected to the right pulmonary artery, and the right pulmonary artery was detached from the main pulmonary artery. Now, the right pulmonary artery is not detached and flow can go to both lung arteries (bidirectional Glenn shunt). The Glenn shunt is placed in patients with single-ventricle anatomy such as hypolastic left- and right-ventricular hearts.

Hybrid Procedure

The hybrid procedure is a new procedure for patients with hypoplastic left heart and is used as an alternative to the modified Norwood procedure. This is a combined invasive cardiac catheterization and closed surgical approach. Via cardiac catheterization, the patent ductus arteriosus (PDA) is stented open, and a balloon atrial septostomy is performed if the atrial communication is restrictive to flow. Via surgery, bilateral pulmonary artery bands are placed to diminish excessive pulmonary blood flow. When the patient is 3-8 months of age, the bidirectional Glenn shunt surgical procedure is performed, along with aortic arch reconstruction if needed. The bands on the pulmonary arteries and the PDA stent are removed.

Kawashima Operation

This intraventricular tunnel repair is used for anatomic correction of double outlet right ventricle where both the aorta and the pulmonary artery originate from the right ventricle and the only exit from the left ventricle is the ventricular septal defect. The ventricular septal defect is left open and sometimes even enlarged to serve as the mouth into a tunnel leading from the left ventricle through the right ventricle to the aorta. This tunnel is called an intracardiac conduit because it occurs completely within the heart. This tunnel is created in such a way as to separate the LV to the aorta and the RV flow to the pulmonary artery. This operation avoids the use of an extracardiac pulmonary conduit.

Ligation (Division) of Patent Ductus Arteriosus

This is one of the truly corrective operations. Once the ductus is successfully closed, no further surgery is required. Ductal closure is a closed-heart procedure consisting of cutting the ductus and sewing up the two stumps. In tiny premature babies, ligation, or tying off, the ductus is preferred, although the ductus frequently reopens.

Mustard Procedure

This procedure, also called a venous switch, is used for physiologic, or functional, correction of transposition of the great arteries (d-transposition). As with a similar procedure, called the Senning operation, the Mustard procedure leaves the transposed origin of the aorta and pulmonary artery unchanged, and instead switches the blood streams entering into the atria. Thus, ultimately, the aorta receives the pink, oxygen-rich blood and the pulmonary artery carries the blue, oxygen-poor blood. This is accomplished by rerouting the blue veins from the right to the left atrium and the pink veins from the left to the right atrium using a partition or "baffle" harvested from the patient's own pericardium, the membranous sac that encloses the heart. The superior vena cava (SVC) and the inferior vena cava (IVC) are directed under the "baffle" into the left atrium (now carrying blue blood), left ventricle and pulmonary artery. The four pulmonary veins flow over the "baffle" into the right atrium,

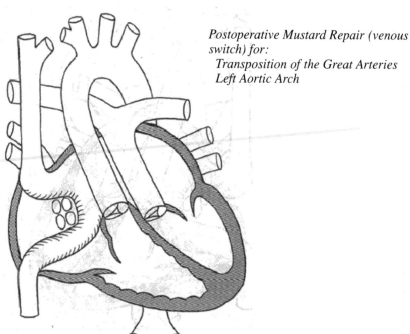

Postoperative Mustard Repair (venous switch) for:
Transposition of the Great Arteries
Left Aortic Arch

which now carries pink blood, and into the right ventricle and aorta. This operation has been, to a large extent, replaced by the arterial switch operation

Norwood Procedures

These procedures are used to treat hypoplastic left heart syndrome, a group of defects in which the left ventricle is very small or absent.

Norwood 1 is a palliative operation—a fix, not a cure—performed in newborns as an emergency procedure using a cardiopulmonary bypass pump. It converts the functional single right ventricle to act as the left ventricle while the pulmonary trunk is surgically joined with the tiny aorta to form a large new aorta, using a modified Damus-Kaye-Stansel procedure. The aortic arch is reconstructed as well, if necessary. The pulmonary artery branches are detached and connected to the new aorta by a small plastic tube, a procedure known as a modified Blalock-Taussig anastomosis. Norwood 1 enables an infant to grow to 4 to 10 months of age, when the second-stage palliative operation can be undertaken.

Norwood 2 converts the Blalock-Taussig anastomosis to a bi-directional Glenn or a Hemi-Fontan anastomosis in preparation for the eventual Fontan procedure, which is the corrective repair. The Glenn and the Hemi-Fontan, a version of the Glenn, consist of connecting both pulmonary artery branches to the superior vena cava, enabling the blue blood to reach the pulmonary circulation directly without having to pass through the heart chambers.

At a suitable age, around 18-24 months, the child becomes eligible for the Fontan operation, which eliminates cyanosis by directing the inferior vena cava to the pulmonary artery and partitioning the two atria.

One-and-One-Half Ventricle Repair

This procedure is used when the right ventricle is too small to handle the entire blue-blood circulation, which ordinarily goes to the lungs for oxygenation. In this operation, the right ventricle is left to pump only the IVC (inferior vena cava) blood to the pulmonary artery, while the SVC (superior vena cava) blood reaches the pulmonary artery through the Glenn anastomosis.

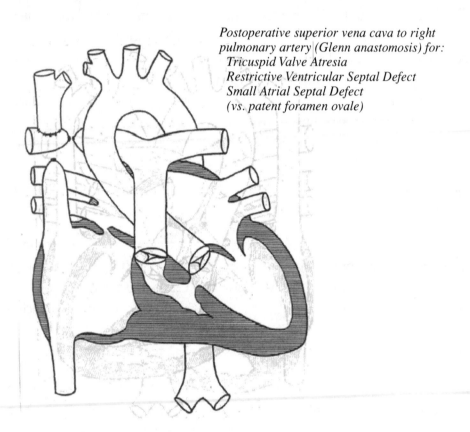

Postoperative superior vena cava to right pulmonary artery (Glenn anastomosis) for:
Tricuspid Valve Atresia
Restrictive Ventricular Septal Defect
Small Atrial Septal Defect
(vs. patent foramen ovale)

Pulmonary Artery Banding

This is a temporary, palliative procedure that reduces excessive flow and pressure in the pulmonary artery. The pulmonary artery is surgically constricted using a wide tape to the point where heart failure due to excessive pulmonary blood flow is controlled. As the child grows, the banded artery remains the same size, causing the child's color to become bluer. At this point a corrective surgery may be carried out, or occasionally, a shunt will be placed to restore the pink color.

Rastelli Procedure

This is an anatomically corrective repair for heart defects that have in common a missing, defective, or obstructed pulmonary artery and a large ventricular septal defect. Truncus arteriosus and transposition of the great arteries, as well as other similar conditions, benefit from the Rastelli procedure.

Basically, the flow of blue blood to the lung circulation is established through a tube placed outside the heart, usually containing a valve. The large ventricular septal defect (VSD) is either closed with a patch or used to construct a new aortic outlet. The valve is placed from the right ventricle to the pulmonary artery. The VSD is closed in such a way as to separate the flow between the ventricles so that the RV flow goes to the pulmonary artery and the LV flow goes solely to the aorta. Such reconstructed hearts have all the components and function of the normal heart. However, the pulmonary conduit cannot grow with the child and eventually requires replacement.

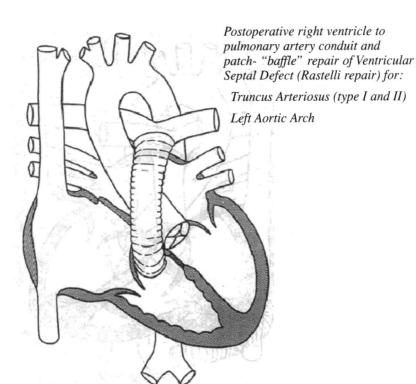

Postoperative right ventricle to pulmonary artery conduit and patch- "baffle" repair of Ventricular Septal Defect (Rastelli repair) for:

Truncus Arteriosus (type I and II)

Left Aortic Arch

Repair of Anomalous Pulmonary Venous Return

Whether some or all four pulmonary veins are draining anomalously into a wrong cardiac structure, the aim of surgery is to re-connect them to the left atrium. If the veins are neither obstructed nor narrow before surgery, the result can be excellent. Obstructed veins, however, tend to re-narrow and may require additional operations.

Repair of Coarctation of the Aorta

This procedure usually does not require cardiopulmonary bypass. A variety of surgical methods are currently in use. Resection, or removal, of the narrowing and an end-to-end anastomosis, a surgical connection of arteries to form a passage, is rarely used because of high recurrence rate. Instead, an extended end-to-end anastomosis offers good long-term repair by removing all the abnormal wall. The subclavian patch repair uses part of the left subclavian artery to enlarge the aortic narrowing, but a plastic patch can be used instead. Rarely is the narrow segment bypassed by a conduit or tube graft.

Repair of Common Atrio-Ventricular (AV) Canal

This anomaly consists of a large confluent atrial and ventricular septal defect and an undivided, or common, inlet valve. Although surgical techniques vary, repair requires patch closure of the two defects and separation of the common valve into a tricuspid and a mitral valve, called the two-ventricle repair. Rarely, when one of the ventricles is too small, a condition called an unbalanced AV canal, a one-ventricle repair, or Fontan operation, is preferable. A partial AV canal, also called an ostium primum defect, consists of a large atrial septal defect and a cleft, or regurgitant, mitral valve. Repair is accomplished by patch closure of the defect and suturing the cleft.

Repair of Tetralogy of Fallot

Tetralogy of Fallot, or blue baby disease, is repaired using a combination of ventricular septal defect closure and repair of narrowings along the pulmonary artery path. An angled patch placed over the large ventricular septal defect serves to channel left ventricular blood into the overriding, or straddling, aorta. Repair of pulmonary stenosis can involve sewing a patch in the right ventricular outflow tract, across the seat of the valve, pulmonary trunk and pulmonary artery branches. When either the pulmonary valve or the trunk is atretic, that is, completely blocked, the Rastelli conduit is required to complete the correction.

When the pulmonary artery is absent, small arteries originating from the aorta called multiple aorta pulmonary collateral arteries, or MAPCAs, supply the lung circulation. This type of tetralogy requires multiple steps to correct. First, MAPCAs on the two sides need to be joined into a single vessel in two separate procedures, called unifocalization. Correction is eventually accomplished using the Rastelli repair.

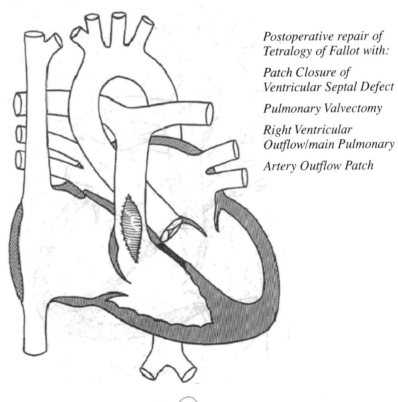

Postoperative repair of Tetralogy of Fallot with:

Patch Closure of Ventricular Septal Defect

Pulmonary Valvectomy

Right Ventricular Outflow/main Pulmonary Artery Outflow Patch

Ross Procedure

This procedure consists of replacing a faulty aortic valve with the patient's own healthy pulmonic valve. It requires re-implantation of the coronary arteries into the reconstructed aortic root. The pulmonic valve is replaced with a bio-logic valve, either homograft taken from a human cadaver donor, or porcine, taken from a pig. This operation can be part of the Ross-Konno procedure employed when there is additional narrowing below the aortic valve. In the Konno procedure, the narrow left ventricular outlet is approached through the right ventricle, the septum is cut open, and filled with a large patch in such a way as to enlarge the LV outflow tract.

Medications

Medications are often required in the treatment of cardiac problems arising from congenital heart defects or surgeries required to correct such defects. Medications do not cure the underlying problem, but may successfully manage the symptoms. The goal of medication treatment is to improve heart function and limit the progression of disease.

There are several categories of cardiac medications used with congenital heart patients, depending on the type of underlying heart problem. This chapter addresses each of these major drug groups. Be sure to consult with your physician, nurse and/or pharmacist for detailed information on any prescribed medication. Carefully note any possible side effects, special considerations and/or warnings.

Always inform any treating doctor or dentist of the complete list of currently prescribed and over-the-counter (OTC) drugs used. Consult your doctor before using most OTC medications or homeopathic/alternative medicine or herbal medicine or vitamins and read all product labels carefully. Many OTC preparations are contraindicated for use with heart or blood pressure problems. There can also be potential drug interactions.

ACE Inhibitors/Vasodilators

Vasodilators are medications that expand or dilate blood vessels and therefore increase blood flow. One of the most frequently used vasodilators is the ACE inhibitor.

ACE stands for angiotensin converting enzyme inhibitor. ACE inhibitors work by blocking the conversion of the enzyme angiotensin I to angiotensin II, which narrows or constricts blood vessels.

ACE inhibitors are used to treat heart failure and hypertension. By reducing vasoconstriction, the vessels' resistance to blood flow, ACE inhibitors help to improve blood flow and in turn can also reduce any congestion of blood in body organs, skin and lungs. By reducing vascular resistance, ACE inhibitors also reduce blood pressure. At the same time, ACE inhibitors also increase renal (kidney) blood flow and therefore have an indirect diuretic effect, removing water from the body through increased urination.

All medications have possible side effects. ACE inhibitors may cause a dry persistent cough, low blood pressure with associated dizziness or weakness and/or swelling of face, lips or neck.

Anticoagulants

Anticoagulants are drugs used to reduce the formation of clots (coagulation) in the blood stream. When the blood is slow to empty from the heart chambers because of poor pumping ability, clots can form and be propelled to lungs or body circulation. Anticoagulants assist in the prevention of stroke, heart attack or pulmonary embolism.

There are three methods of administering anticoagulants. Heparin is administered via intravenous lines, which is helpful when it is necessary to provide immediate anticoagulant protection. Lovenox, an injectable form, is often used when first beginning anticoagulant therapy because it is faster than the oral method. Oral therapy is used for long-term effects, usually as the medication warfarin (Coumadin). Low-dose aspirin therapy is used for gentler anticoagulation.

When taking oral anticoagulants, the prescribing physician will schedule regular blood testing called prothrombin time or INR test (international normalized ratio) to monitor therapeutic blood clotting times. This is to ensure that the blood is not "too thin," meaning too anticoagulated, or "too thick," meaning not anticoagulated enough. There is a desired therapeutic range, which may vary slightly depending on the heart problem being treated. Patients on anticoagulation medication may need adjustment or interruption of treatment before dental or surgical procedures.

Vitamin K helps the blood make clots. While on anticoagulant medication, a child does not need to avoid these types of food, but parents should take care to keep them at a consistent level in the diet. Leafy green vegetables are very high in vitamin K.

Anticoagulants are very important medications. If not taken properly, or not regularly monitored, they can cause serious complications, such as uncontrolled bleeding. There are several special considerations for patients who are taking anticoagulant medications.

Timing. It is important to take this medicine at the same time each day. If a dose is accidentally omitted, do not double the next dose.

Interactions. This medication can have significant interactions with other medications. Consult with your doctor before adding any new medicine, even over-the-counter medicines—such as aspirin or ibuprofen. Be sure to inform any physician or dentist that your child is taking warfarin/Coumadin and why.

Alcohol. Warfarin/Coumadin's effect can be exaggerated by the use of alcohol, which may increase the risk of bleeding problems.

Contact sports. Contact sports, such as boxing, hockey and football, should be avoided during the use of anticoagulants.

Head trauma or headache. If your child experiences significant head trauma, or unusual headache, inform your doctor immediately.

Abnormal bleeding. If any abnormal bleeding is observed, consult your physician immediately. For example: bleeding that does not stop easily, blood in urine or stool, vomiting blood or coffee ground-like material, coughing up blood, or excessive bruising.

Medi-alert bracelet. It is advisable for your child to wear a medi-alert bracelet, neck chain pendant or wallet card stating the use of warfarin/Coumadin, in the event you are unable to communicate to emergency professionals.

Stay informed. Talk with your doctor, nurse or pharmacist about receiving literature on anticoagulant medicines.

Antiarrhythmics

There are several types of drugs used to treat irregular heartbeats, or arrhythmias. These medications act on specific sites to alter the transmission of electrical impulses that signal the heart to beat.

Amiodarone. Amiodarone is used to treat recurrent ventricular fibrillation, unstable ventricular tachycardia, supraventricular arrhythmias and atrial fibrillation. Amiodarone has diverse effects on several sites in the heart to suppress abnormal signal formation and conduction. It is among the most commonly used agents to control irregular heart rhythms. Patients who take amiodarone must be monitored for four main potential side effects: pulmonary fibrosis by chest x-ray and pulmonary function tests; thyroid function laboratory tests to look for thyroid dysfunction; liver function lab test to monitor for liver toxicity; and, regular eye exams to monitor for optic neuropathy.

Parents are advised to make sure their child wears sunscreen because of increased risk of photosensitivity, especially sunburn and blistering, when taking amiodarone. Parents may also be encouraged to give their child this medication with meals to avoid stomach upset. The potential for drug/drug interactions, especially with digoxin and dilantin, may require the prescribing doctor to readjust other medication doses.

Adenosine. Adenosine is used to treat paroxysmal supraventricular tachycardia. It acts on the atrio-ventricular node to slow conduction. This drug is only available in intravenous form and is therefore only administered in the hospital setting. It is to be used with caution in patients with asthma because it may cause bronchospasm.

Beta blockers. Beta blockers are used to treat arrhythmias by prolonging the refractory period (nonexcitable) of the AV node and reducing AV conduction, thereby reducing the likelihood that extra beats will occur. (See below for more in Beta Blockers.)

Calcium channel blockers. Calcium channel blockers act to reduce calcium influx into the cells, especially at the SA and AV nodes, thereby slowing conduction through the heart. They are used to slow the ventricular rate in atrial fibrillation or flutter and to convert supraventricular tachycardia to normal rhythm.

Digoxin. (See Inotropic Drugs below.)

Beta Blockers

Beta blockers are used to treat a variety of medical problems from hypertension, angina, arrhythmias, heart failure, and myocardial infarct to migraine headaches and benign tremors.

In the treatment of hypertension, beta blockers are thought to reduce cardiac output, decrease the release of the kidney hormone renin, and lower the sympathetic effect on the central nervous system that results in excitability of the heart muscle. In anginal treatment, beta blockers decrease the heart muscle's oxygen demands by blocking increases in heart rate, blood pressure and heart contraction induced by catecholamine or adrenaline.

Beta blockers used to treat arrhythmias act to prolong the refractory (nonexcitable) period of the AV (atrio-ventricular) node and reduce AV conduction, thereby reducing the likelihood that extra beats or palpitations will occur.

For patients at risk of myocardial infarction, some beta blockers are used to prevent a heart attack. The mechanism responsible is not yet fully understood.

Possible side effects of beta blocker medications include: low heart rate, fatigue, depression, insomnia, nightmares, memory loss and impotence. These medications can affect blood sugars and should be used with caution in diabetic patients. These medications are not recommended for patients with asthma as they can exaggerate bronchospasm.

As with all prescription medications, beta blockers should be taken as directed on a regular schedule and not abruptly discontinued unless advised by the prescribing physician.

Be sure to consult your doctor before taking any new medication to avoid possible drug interactions.

Diuretics

Diuretics are often referred to as "water pills" because they stimulate the kidneys to remove excess water and salt from the body by increased urine output. There are several types of diuretics and they all have the same main effect, but act upon various parts of the kidneys.

Diuretics are used in the treatment of heart failure and hypertension. They are often used in combination with other medications. Some diuretics can lead to potassium depletion and a potassium supplement may be prescribed. However, not all diuretics cause potassium loss. Some are potassium sparing. It is advisable to take diuretics in the morning so the majority of diuresis (urination) will occur before bedtime. The physician may ask patients to keep a log of their daily weights to monitor the diuretic effect and therefore control of heart failure to avoid potential dehydration.

Experimental Drugs/Drug Studies

Medical researchers make gains everyday in the discovery of new treatments. Before new medications can be approved by the FDA, they must be rigorously studied, first on animals and then on people. There may be benefits to being enrolled in a drug study. The medicine is usually available to patients free of charge along with free medical follow-up. However, you must first be sure that the research is being conducted by a reputable hospital, university and physician. You may contact the FDA office of consumer affairs to find out more about experimental drug studies.

Inotropic Drugs

The inotropic, or muscle strengthening, medications, such as digoxin are prescribed for the treatment of heart failure, atrial fibrillation or flutter, or paroxysmal atrial tachycardia.

In heart failure, digoxin causes the heart to slow down and pump blood more efficiently. It increases cardiac output by increasing the force of each contraction of the heart muscle (systole).

Digoxin is used to treat rapid heart rates because of its ability to increase the parasympathetic nervous system, thereby counteracting excess catecholamine activity produced by heart failure. Digoxin may be used alone or in combination with other medications.

Side effects include nausea, vomiting, visual changes and fatigue especially if there is too much Digoxin in the system (digoxin toxicity).

It is advisable to take digoxin at a regular time each day and consult your doctor before taking any new medicines.

There are other inotropic (muscle strengthening) medications such as dobutamine and dopamine, which are more potent but only available in IV form. Their action is dose dependent, which means low doses and high doses will cause different actions. These are only administered in the hospital.

Potassium Supplements
Potassium supplements are sometimes prescribed in conjunction with some diuretics because of an increased loss of potassium with the extra fluid loss. A balance of potassium is necessary for the proper function of the heart's electrical impulses. Significantly high or low potassium can cause irregular heartbeats. Potassium levels can be measured by a simple blood chemistry test.

In addition, a diet rich in potassium, found in bananas, orange juice, carrot juice, is often recommended.

Conclusion
This chapter has briefly touched on several categories of medications. Additional detailed medication information is available from physicians, nurses, and pharmacists. Always inform any treating doctor or dentist of the complete list of prescribed and over-the-counter medications being taken. Consult with your doctor before using most over-the-counter medications or homeopathic/alternative medicines. Be advised to read all product labels carefully.

Congenital Heart Disease in the Adult

General Issues

There are now more people over the age of 18 living with congenital heart defects (CHDs) than there are people under the age of 18. Since the advent of the heart-lung machine in the 1950s, many additional technological and surgical advances have been made available allowing over 90 percent of the children born with CHDs to survive well into adulthood. Thanks to these increases in survival, the number of adults with CHDs continues to rise at a rate of approximately 5% a year.

According to the Adult Congenital Heart Association, there are about one million adults and 800,000 children in the U.S. living with congenital heart defects. Government statistics show that approximately 40,000 babies are born each year with a CHD, one out of every 125 births. Unfortunately these statistics only show the number of babies identified with a CHD. There are at least an additional 10% who are born with a CHD that go undetected until adulthood.

For Those Transitioning from Childhood to Adulthood

The age a person with a CHD starts living as an adult, with less influence from their parents, doesn't magically happen at age 18. For some it can be earlier, for others later. The key is to make sure you start talking with your pediatric cardiologist about life-long follow-up care before you leave the care of your parents. This conversation may feel scary for a person who has had a relationship with a particular cardiologist since birth. As an adult, however, it's always good to consider a consultation with an adult cardiologist who has sub-specialty training in congenital heart disease. They will be looking at your heart defect with a focus of how it might be impacted by regular heart disease as well as the normal wear and tear of the heart defect and/or repair itself. Whether you initiate the conversation or your pediatric cardiologist does, it is important for you to have a copy of your medical records, including a DVD of your last heart scan. Continuity of care is important to your longevity and quality of life. The Children's Heart Foundation recommends that you not let more than a year go by without seeing a CHD specialist during this transition period.

If you no longer have contact with your pediatric cardiologist, seek out a consultation with a trained adult congenital heart specialist in your city or region. There are thousands of CHD patients who were told after surgery that their heart defects were fixed when in reality they were just repaired. The long-term health issues that might affect your heart could shorten your lifespan if left undiagnosed too long later in life.

For Adults

If you were born with a congenital heart defect, you become an adult with a congenital heart defect. People with CHDs need life-long monitoring by a trained cardiologist. If you have had any kind of repair on your heart, you should be looking for a cardiologist who has formal training in congenital heart disease. A general adult cardiologist may not fully understand how your CHD affects the heart when an acquired heart disease issue arises. It is important in all cases to keep a copy of your medical records updated.

Surgery can repair the defects, but it doesn't necessarily permanently correct the defect. May times additional repairs are needed to replace valves, stents, and conduits. Functional capacity can change, arrhythmias can develop and classic or subtle cardiac symptoms will need to be brought to your doctor's attention. Congenital heart defects have moved from the number-one birth defect in the U.S. to also becoming a major chronic illness that requires life-long specialized care.

Congenital heart disease is different from "regular" or "acquired" heart problems. Not all cardiologists are familiar with the different types of congenital heart disease. Don't be afraid to ask questions or to ask for a consultation with a congenital heart specialist if you were born with or think you might have a congenital heart defect.

In 2010, the American College of Cardiology and the American Academy of

Pediatrics announced the creation on a new subspecialty in congenital heart disease for adult cardiologists. There are over 150 medical centers throughout the U.S. that have congenital heart programs. To find a center near you, contact the Adult Congenital Heart Association or the American College of Cardiology.

Know What Your Heart Defect Is

You are unique and so is your congenital heart defect. Like snowflakes, no two are alike. It is important to know what your heart defect is and what medical treatments you have had. If you have a CHD, it is important to see your cardiologist on a regular basis. Subtle changes can turn into big, life threatening problems that could have been prevented if you had been seeing a cardiac specialist.

Longevity and quality of life have become the new focus for many in the congenital heart world. Research and clinical trials are being conducted at select CHD centers throughout the U.S. and Canada to find better ways to care for patients early on in a effort to minimize neurological issues that seem to be more prevalent in children with some complex congenital heart defects.

Clinical trials and research studies can provide patients a space to become more active participants in their medical care. Participating in these trials also helps the congenital heart community as a whole. If you are interested in participating in a study on congenital heart defects, contact your CHD specialist or the National Heart, Blood and Lung Institute at the National Institutes of Health.

Patient Registry and Surveillance System

Before 2010, there were no national CHD patient registries. Collecting basic data on incidence, morbidity, mortality and outcomes of the various surgical procedures for CHD repair were kept by the individual institutions.

In 2010, The American College of Cardiology launched their pilot for a national clinical data registry that will enroll pediatric and adult patients who undergo cardiac catheterization. The registry is called The IMPACT Registry— short for Improved Pediatric and Adult Congenital Treatment. Its goal is to focus on episodes of care that will provide a collection of data that hopefully will not only improve care around surgery or catheterization, but over the lifetime of the individual.

With the enactment of health care reform by Congress in 2010, the Congenital Heart Futures Act became law. The law specifies that the National Institutes of Health (NIH) conduct congenital heart defect research across the lifespan and that the Centers for Disease Control (CDC) create a National Congenital Heart Surveillance System (NCHSS). Even thought the Futures Act is now law, funding has yet to be appropriated. To learn more about this important program, go to The Children's Heart Foundation website.

Preventive Measures for Healthy Lifestyle

Developing healthy habits that will continue throughout one's life is key for everyone, but especially for adults born with CHD. Healthy habits improve one's general well being as well as help prevent heart attack, stroke, high blood pressure, diabetes, and some cancers. Developing cardiovascular fitness can help reduce the extra stress on the heart and lungs from the original heart disease and subsequent surgeries. Recommendations for developing a healthier lifestyle include:

1. **Don't smoke tobacco/minimize exposure to secondhand smoke.** Smoking limits the amount of oxygen going to the body tissues, increases heart rate and blood pressure, increases the risk of developing blood clots, and damages arteries throughout the body, but especially in the heart and brain. In addition, smoking increases the risk for various lung diseases, of extra concern for persons with cyanotic heart disease.

Second-hand smoke exposure (environmental tobacco smoke) is also a serious health hazard. It increases a non-smoker's risk of death from heart disease and lung cancer and, in children living with an adult who smokes at home, it increases susceptibility to various illnesses.

The addictive effects of nicotine often make it very difficult to quit smoking once one starts; therefore, every effort should be made not to start smoking. If an adult with CHD already smokes, the most important thing to do to improve health is to quit. A variety of resources are available from health care professionals, the American Heart Association (AHA), and the American Cancer Society to help stop smoking.

2. Eat a healthy diet. Aim for a diet that is low in fat and cholesterol and high in fiber. This type of diet is recommended by the AHA and other groups to help prevent heart disease and stroke as well as some cancers. For the American public in general, the AHA recommends a diet that limits fat intake to about 30% of total calories (called the AHA Step I Diet). (The average American currently consumes about 40% of total calories from fat.) Get into the habit of reading food labels to find the fat content of food products and go easy on those high in saturated fat or cholesterol.

Limit salt intake. This is of special concern for people with high blood pressure or heart failure.

3. Maintain a healthy weight. Extra weight causes extra work for the heart. Losing weight can help reduce this excess stress and, in addition, help control blood pressure and cholesterol levels, and decrease the chance of developing diabetes. Two recommended methods to estimate body fat are waist circumference and body mass index (BMI). Females with a waist greater than 35 inches and males with a waist greater than 40 inches are considered at greater risk for cardiac and vascular disease. Body mass index (determined from a person's height and weight) categorizes body fat as follows:

- $18.5\text{-}24$ kg/m^2 = "healthy"

- $25\text{-}29$ kg/m^2 = "overweight" (about 10% over ideal)

- 30 kg/m^2 or greater = "obese" (greater than 30 pounds over ideal weight).

BMI tables can be found at physician offices, on many web sites and in books about obesity and/or weight loss. One quick calculation for adults is shown below:

FEMALES: Baseline = 100 lbs.; add 5 lbs. for every inch over 5 ft.

Example: 5'4" female = 100 + 20 (additional 4 in. x 5 lbs.) = 120 lbs.

MALES: Baseline = 110 lbs.; add 6 lbs. for every inch over 5 ft.

Example: 6'1" male = 110 + 78 (additional 13 in. x 6 lbs.) = 188 lbs.

4. Exercise regularly. A regular exercise program is encouraged for everyone. While exercise can improve the way one looks and feels, it also has other benefits:

- Helps lower blood pressure and resting heart rate; it can also improve blood flow to the heart.
- Allows the heart to do work with less energy.
- Helps increase HDL or the "good" cholesterol level in the blood.
- Improves flexibility of the muscles and joints, building muscle strength and tone.
- Along with a proper diet, aids in weight loss.
- Relieves stress and tension—helps relax the body and improves sleep.

The AHA recommends 30-60 minutes of aerobic activity (walking, jogging, swimming, etc.) at least 4 times a week for cardiovascular fitness. The need for individualized restrictions should be discussed with your physician. (*Refer to the section: Activity/Exercise*). Many individuals with CHD had their activity restricted in childhood and may need extra encouragement as adults to exercise on a routine basis.

5. Know your cholesterol. Monitor your cholesterol and know if high cholesterol is in your family history. High blood cholesterol levels, especially LDL-cholesterol (the "bad" cholesterol), are well known to increase one's risk of coronary heart disease. The National Cholesterol Education Program recommends that everyone over 20 years old get their cholesterol checked at least every five years. Cholesterol levels can be lowered by a diet low in fat and cholesterol and by an appropriate exercise program. Some people will require lipid-lowering medication, along with diet and exercise.

6. Know your blood pressure. Monitor your blood pressure and know if high blood pressure is in your family history. A blood pressure reading measures the force of blood as it presses against the walls of the blood vessels and is made up of two numbers: 1) the top number or systolic blood pressure measures the force while the heart pumps, and 2) the bottom number or diastolic blood pressure measures the force while the heart is at rest. High blood pressure or hypertension is defined as a systolic pressure of 140 or greater and/or a diastolic pressure of 90 or greater.

7. If high blood pressure is or has been a problem… Focus on lifestyle measures to ensure that your blood pressure stays within the normal range. High blood pressure puts extra work on the heart. It is important that you follow your physician's advice on losing weight, cutting down on salt, exercising, taking needed medicines, quitting smoking, and reducing stress. Since high blood pressure often goes undetected, it is important to have it checked periodically.

8. Know your family history of heart disease. It's important to know your family's history of both congenital and acquired (e.g., heart attack, heart failure, angina, etc.) heart disease. Predisposition to a variety of problems tends to run in families. It is important that every individual knows his or her family history as physicians may institute special preventive measures to help those at high risk for acquired heart disease. Some inherited problems may require further family testing.

9. Consult your physician for advice on intake of alcohol. Because drinking alcohol has varying effects on the body, as well as interactions with certain medications, you should consult your physician for specific recommendations. Pregnant women should not drink alcohol in any form as it can cause the baby serious harm, including birth defects. Excessive consumption of alcohol has direct effects on the heart, as well as other important body organs, weakening the heart's muscle and its ability to pump adequately.

10. Avoid illicit drugs. Most of these drugs have very dangerous effects on the heart and should especially be avoided in persons with a pre-existing heart problem. Dangerously rapid cardiac rhythms, cardiac arrest, heart attack, and abnormalities in blood pressure are some of the effects noted in the cardiovascular system. In addition, intravenous drug use provides another route for bacteria to enter the bloodstream and produce a dangerous infection within the heart called endocarditis.

Activity/Exercise

Although some adults born with CHD may be subjected to varying physical limitations regarding exercise, many will have no restrictions. Restrictions are dependent on the type of CHD, the success of the repair, the current physical condition of the individual and current medications being taken.

Overall, individuals should look for activities that keep the heart and lungs fit as well as ones that are enjoyable. For maximum benefit of the heart and lungs, exercise should be rhythmic and aerobic (exercising at an intensity where oxygen is used for energy). Examples of aerobic activities are brisk walking, jogging, recreational cycling, swimming, and low impact aerobics. Higher levels of intensity are associated with anaerobic activity, which is more stressful to the cardiovascular system and should have a cardiologist's approval.

In addition, activities to improve strength and flexibility (e.g., stretching exercises) should be incorporated into one's fitness program. Some individuals with CHD may be restricted from activities that are highly strenuous, i.e., have a large proportion of "isometric" muscle movement. Examples of these activities include heavy weight-lifting or pushing heavy pieces of furniture. Increase in blood pressure, which stresses the heart and the aorta, is greater with isometric exercise than with aerobic activities.

Key factors that are considered in determining the best exercise program for each individual include:

1. **What is the intensity of the activity—low, moderate, or high?** For example, brisk walking or social dancing are usually described as "moderate," while running or vigorous biking are usually considered "high" intensity activities. The appropriate intensity is often determined by the peak heart rate and blood pressure that the individual reaches during a treadmill stress test.

2. **What will be the duration & frequency of the activity?** The minimum effective duration of cardiovascular workout is 15-20 minutes, with a goal being 30-60 minutes and a frequency of 3-5 times/week.

3. **What will be the risk of body collision during the sport or activity?** This is often an area of concern to children and adults taking anticoagulants, or who have a pacemaker, or who have Marfan's syndrome. Hockey, soccer, and football are examples of activities that are considered high risk for body collision.

4. **Will the activity be competitive (usually vigorous, approached with higher intensity), recreational (for pleasure and relaxation, usually more self-limiting), or restricted (prescribed amount)?**

5. **What kind of training or conditioning is required?**

6. **What will be the emotional response (or stress) that the participant experiences in anticipation of or during the event?**

7. **What are the environmental conditions associated with the activity?** For example, individuals need to consider extremely cold or warm temperatures and the effects of high altitude.

Every adult with a history of CHD should seek approval and recommendations from his or her cardiologist. Most will need to undergo a basic stress test at intervals to evaluate the heart's response to exercise—especially if there has been a recent change in health and/or a new exercise program is being undertaken. Occasionally, more sophisticated stress testing may be recommended.

Preventing Endocarditis

(See Chapter Nine for more on SBE prophylaxis.)

Dental Care

As in childhood, good dental hygiene habits should be maintained to prevent bacteria from entering the bloodstream and causing a life-threatening heart infection. Dental visits for cleaning and checkups are recommended at least every six months. Dentists should be kept up-to-date of any changes in your heart condition and/or medications, especially blood thinners, such as Coumadin.

Some individuals with a congenital heart defect have been advised to take antibiotics before dental procedures; they should continue this practice even after surgical repair unless counseled otherwise by their cardiologists. Recommendations for antibiotic use (issued jointly by the American Heart Association and the American Dental Association) change from time to time —if any questions arise, your cardiologist should always be contacted for clarification.

In addition to routine checkups, adults with heart problems should continue brushing with a soft toothbrush twice daily, once in the morning and again before going to bed. You should also floss carefully once a day, taking care not to traumatize the gums. Check with your dentist or physician if your gums bleed excessively, especially if you are taking blood thinners.

Skin Care

It is important to remember that the skin provides a "barrier" against potentially serious infections – an especially important barrier if you have CHD. Anything that could break this barrier should be avoided, such as picking at cuticles, scabs, or pimples. A dermatologist should be consulted for possible antibiotic treatment of severe acne.

Questions regarding tattoos, body piercing, or electrolysis should be discussed with your cardiologist. If it is approved, prophylactic antibiotics may be advised. Before the procedure, the skin should be thoroughly washed; after the procedure, any sign of redness, swelling or discharge should be noted and reported to one's primary physician immediately!

Regularly Established Plan for Follow-up of Heart Problem

It is important to develop a plan for general health maintenance and follow-up of CHD as teens/young adults leave home and/or the care of their pediatrician. It is often at this point that many adults do not continue with follow-up medical care. Inadequate health care coverage as an adult may be a contributing factor. (See section on Insurability.) Women may follow up with their obstetrician/gynecologist, who may, in turn, refer them to an adult cardiologist, especially in the case of pregnancy. (See section on Reproductive Issues.)

Follow-up care includes a physical examination with intermittent echocardiograms and/or exercise stress tests by a cardiologist who specializes in the care of patients with CHD. The visit should include time for discussion about the various topics introduced in this chapter, e.g., recommendations regarding exercise, insurance issues, problems with employment, sexual concerns, family planning issues, and clarifying information about heart problems, medications, etc.

Any time individuals change residence and/or change cardiologists, they should obtain a copy of their medical records to take with them to the new appointment. This should include catheterizations, operations, and recent echocardiograms and ECGs (electrocardiograms).

Hospitalization and/or ER Visit

Adults with CHD may need to be seen in a hospital, clinic, doctor's office, or emergency room in which the staff may be unfamiliar with the care of congenital heart problems. An unexpected hospitalization, an emergency non-cardiac surgery or treatment of trauma can be much riskier for the CHD patient. It is your responsibility to be knowledgeable about your heart condition. Carry an abbreviated medical history, including dates and types of surgeries, a list of current medications (with dose and when taken), the need for antibiotic prophylaxis, and the name and telephone number of the cardiologist whenever possible. A MedicAlert bracelet or neck pendant should also be considered for specific problems and telephone numbers.

In the event of a non-cardiac procedure, CHD patients should first receive clearance from their cardiologists. Most people will tolerate non-cardiac procedures well. Certain individuals with higher risk of cardiac complication (e.g., patients with cyanotic heart problems, heart failure, or heart rhythm abnormalities) will require careful monitoring during the procedure and special considerations when the anesthesia is administered. This may mean having the procedure done at a specialized center and/or with specific recommendations from a congenital heart specialist. In addition, special precautions may need to be taken before or during the procedure if the person has a pacemaker or implantable defibrillator. The device may need to be double-checked after the procedure to make sure that the settings were not affected by any electrical interference. After surgery, getting out of bed and walking as early as possible will be especially important to prevent blood clots from developing.

Travel Considerations

The need to restrict travel depends on the type of CHD and the individual's current overall health status. When selecting a destination, the following factors should be considered:

1. Access to emergency medical care. Inquire where and what type of emergency care is available and where a person would be taken for advanced care and hospitalization. A letter with current medical information should be carried at all times. (See section on Hospitalization.)

2. Physical stress associated with the itinerary. Some destinations require much walking and climbing and/or very long, tiring days. Whenever possible, modify your schedule to lessen unnecessary physical stress.

3. The extremes of altitude and climate, especially high altitudes (e.g., ski trips) and extreme heat or cold:

   • High altitude: It may be worthwhile to take the first few days of the trip to get acclimated to the altitude – the "thinner air" and less available oxygen– before starting with rigorous physical activity/touring.

- Extreme heat: In this situation it is important to keep activity at a "reasonable" minimum and drink enough fluids to stay hydrated. Water is the fluid of choice and should be kept available at all times. Alcohol should be avoided because it can, among other things, cause further loss of body fluid.

- Extreme cold: Out-of-doors activity may need to be restricted in this type of climate (including shoveling snow). Cold temperatures cause blood vessels to constrict, thus forcing the heart to work harder to get blood through the narrower vessels.

For the various situations encountered when traveling, adults with CHD should be prudent and use common sense, but not live in fear that they should needlessly restrict their lifestyle. Any questions or concerns should be directed to your cardiologist.

Patients with pulmonary hypertension, cyanotic heart disease, and severe heart failure are at risk at high altitude and during air travel. They should not travel in mountainous areas significantly higher than 5,000 feet (e.g., Denver, Mexico City). When flying, supplemental oxygen may be required. The airlines need to be notified of this special request in advance – an extra charge will be incurred. When traveling by air, especially on long flights, individuals should be encouraged to frequently get up and move about the cabin. This keeps blood from pooling in the legs and feet and forming blood clots.

Lifestyle Issues
Employability

One of the important life decisions for adults born with CHD is choice of career path. Start talking about careers early on, beginning in junior and senior high schools. Choices should be realistic for one's mental, physical, and social or personal abilities. Although most individuals with CHD enter the workforce with unlimited restrictions, many young adults with complex defects develop physical limitations as they get older. When evaluating career opportunities, the major focus should be to look at an area where a person can potentially work through to retirement, even with increasing physical limitations. Discuss questions and concerns with the cardiologist. The document "Occupational Recommendations for Young Patients with Heart Disease" (AHA, 1986) may provide additional information for those seeking advice. State-run vocational rehabilitation services are available and provide vocational counseling and training for those identified with either a physical or mental disability.

Adults with CHD may experience workplace discrimination once they pursue a job. Discrimination may be felt to varying degrees and may be attributed to uncertainty about physical ability, fear of absenteeism due to illness or doctors' appointments, and the rising costs of providing insurance benefits. If you feel that you are being treated unfairly by your employer because of CHD, you may have rights under the ADA (Americans with Disabilities Act) and various state laws. However, disability discrimination involves a complicated analysis of the medical condition, as well as the work circumstances. Be sure to seek competent legal advice before initiating a complaint or legal action to determine the best approach for your particular problem. The EEOC (Equal Employment Opportunity Commission) does accept these charges and will assist an individual in writing the charge, but that does not guarantee that the EEOC will act on the charge and prosecute the claim. Prompt attention to the problem at work when it starts is essential, because delay can result in denial of legal redress or cause the problems to persist at work and get worse.

A list of other federal government resources for which persons with disabilities may be eligible can be obtained from the U.S. Department of Education.

Insurability

Health insurance coverage often becomes an issue in late teens or early 20s. Before this time, a child with CHD will be covered on his or her parent's policy or is covered through a state-funded health program. The best way to obtain coverage is through one's job or the job of a family member. The Health Insurance Portability and Accountability Act of 1997 eliminated the 12-month waiting period often imposed when switching health plans. Now this waiting period only applies to those with a pre-existing condition and no health insurance for the previous 12 months (e.g., those coming out from under parent's policy). Young adults can often work around this by planning needed follow-up care before leaving their parent's policy or after the 12-month wait. When changing jobs, evaluate insurance options and try to avoid letting coverage lapse. Continuing coverage under COBRA (Combined Omnibus Budget Reconciliation Act) during extended times of unemployment should be pursued before leaving a current employer.

The following points should be considered when obtaining insurance for health care:

- Seek employment with a large company (likely to offer generous health benefit packages).

- Check for restrictions (e.g., special waiting periods).

- Look for ways to cut coverage (increase deductibles, etc.).

- Check structure of plan. (Some companies are self-insured. Pay special attention to how the plans are structured and administered.)

- Get dental coverage if possible.

- See if the plan handles prescription drugs.

- Examine if there would be difficulty obtaining referrals for specialist care (e.g., cardiologist with adult congenital heart disease focus).

Request that a medical person from the insurance company review your case, as nonmedical insurance personnel will more often reject your insurance inquiry due to lack of medical knowledge. Some states have enacted legislation creating a risk-sharing or reinsurance pooling for otherwise "medically uninsurable" individuals. Unfortunately, these programs also carry higher premiums. Because eligibility varies from state to state, specific information can be obtained by contacting each state's insurance board.

Adults who are unemployed or who have insufficient income may qualify for coverage under Medicaid. This jointly-funded federal-state health insurance program includes coverage for physician visits and hospitalizations. Application is usually made at the state Department of Human Services office. If the cost of medications becomes a hardship, many drug companies have programs for the indigent which can be pursued through your physician's office or through a very comprehensive listing at the website www.needymeds.com.

Unfortunately, there are still many individuals unable to qualify for Medicaid who are among the working poor and lower-middle class (often seasonal workers, short-term employment at low wages). These people usually have no health insurance and find long-term health care difficult to obtain. They may want to explore county or state medical providers or local clinics funded by special grants—including those also offering dental care. Ultimately, these individuals should consider vocational counseling and/or job training and search for employment in areas with better insurance coverage and more stable employment.

Life Insurance

Life insurance is desirable as a means of establishing financial independence for you and your family. Although more liberal coverage is available today, adults with congenital heart disease remain underinsured, compared with the general population. Not enough is known about the lifespan of individuals who had their defects repaired 20-30 years ago. Therefore insurance companies have very old information on which to base the insurability risk for certain congenital conditions. Individuals having difficulty obtaining life insurance may want to pursue some of the following options:

- If turned down as a child, try at a later time, especially after 16 years of age.

- Seek assistance from your personal physician to provide supportive information, interpret test results, etc.

- Try large well-known companies; sign up when starting a new job.

- Shop around; try an independent insurance agent who usually works with several companies with different restrictions.

- Consider group term life insurance.

- Try to build equity other than through life insurance.

Request that a medical person from the insurance company review your case, as nonmedical insurance personnel will more often reject your insurance inquiry due to lack of medical knowledge.

Psychosocial Issues

Most young people who have grown up with the diagnosis of CHD and the associated stressful experiences (e.g., major surgery, multiple doctor visits, restricted physical activities) appear to have adjusted well and have few behavioral issues as they move into adulthood. In fact, these individuals often show an amazing ability to cope with stress later on in life, attributed to their encounters with stressful experiences in the earlier years.

On the other hand, because of problems experienced in childhood, individuals with CHD may develop some of the following problems in adjustment as they move into their adult years:

Accepting one's illness as an adult:

Depending on the diagnosis, some people with CHD may be faced with new limitations or changes in their condition as they enter the adult years, forcing them to take a hard look at their illness and life goals. Support from family and friends can be extremely important.

Anxiety and depression:

Both anxiety and depression appear more frequently in adults with CHD than in the general population. Both can be treated if recognized and appropriate help is sought. Bring these issues up for discussion with your congenital heart physician. The cardiologist may refer you to a psychologist or psychiatrist, ideally one who has a close working relationship with the cardiologist to make consultation easier for medications and other aspects of care.

Family and friends can help with behavioral issues. Your congenital heart physician can also help. Do not be afraid to bring these issues up at any doctor's visit. Adults with CHD may also find it helpful to locate others with like issues for support and discussion. Most major cities have support groups for adults with congenital heart problems and several web sites run by adults with similar problems can be found on the internet.

Developing non-compliant, destructive behaviors:

Some adolescents and young adults don't accept their illness or minimize its importance up to the point of feeling incapable of experiencing any harm. They stop taking their medications or seeing their physician for follow-up. Some get involved with destructive behaviors, like alcohol or drugs. The difficult task of getting to the root of these behaviors is necessary to prevent persons from doing permanent harm to themselves and putting additional stress on their heart. Education regarding abusive behavior should begin very early.

Difficulty in developing independence:

Some individuals with CHD remain in a very passive, dependent role as they become adults, relinquishing the adult role to others (e.g., parents, physician, or spouse). Often this problem is associated with pampering and overprotection during childhood. Along with fostering independence in general, parents must assure that adolescents/young adults start taking responsibility for their own healthcare—knowing all about their congenital problem, past surgeries and hospitalizations, and medications. (See General Health Care Issues: Plan for Follow-up Care & Hospitalization and/or ER Visit). As individuals with CHD move through the teen years, they should start visiting with the doctor alone and be assisted in transitioning to adult physicians.

Sexual/marital concerns:

Concerns often arise as young people with CHD begin dating. They may not know when to disclose that they have a "heart problem," and perhaps hesitate saying anything at all for fear of rejection. There is typically more expressed concern over sexual issues than with other chronic diseases—by both young men and women—such as fear of performance or of dying in bed. CHD can be accompanied by problems of low esteem, resulting in a need to limit romantic aspirations or seek relationships with people who are "caretakers." Additional concerns arising with marriage include feelings of uncertainty over the financial provider role, and for women, their childbearing ability. (See section on Reproductive Issues). Ask your cardiologist about sexual issues, including sexual orientation. It is important to get needed information and referral to appropriate resources.

Workplace issues:

Within the workplace, CHD adults may face real or perceived disadvantages in the job market and with job discrimination. (See section on Employability).

Reproductive Issues
Menarche & Menstruation

In general, young women with CHD have their first menstrual period (the ability to ovulate and conceive) later than the "average" age of 12.3 years in the general population. Girls with acyanotic (pink) heart defects begin their periods slightly later than the general population, but then tend to have fairly normal menstrual patterns. Girls with cyanotic (blue) heart problems begin their menstrual periods significantly later and tend to experience more irregularities, such as break-through bleeding and missed periods.

If a woman with CHD needs to be started on any medications to regulate her period, she should first consult with her cardiologist (congenital heart disease doctor).

Birth Control

Discussions on birth control and any risk from pregnancy should be initiated in early adolescence, especially for women in whom pregnancy could cause major cardiac problems or be life threatening. (See section on Pregnancy.)

The appropriate type of birth control for women born with CHD varies widely, depending on the type of heart problem and its repair:

- *Barrier methods* (e.g., sponge, diaphragm, condom) are about 80% reliable if used correctly with spermicide; this is improved if the male uses a condom at the same time that the female uses a barrier. Barrier methods are very safe and are often recommended for the woman with CHD.

- *Oral contraceptives* (especially estrogen/progestin combination) are very effective (97% reliable) but may be problematic for some women as they are associated with blood pressure problems, salt and water retention, and blood clotting risks.

- *Long-acting intradermal preparations* (such as Norplant/methylprogestin) are highly effective as above. This type of contraceptive may be an acceptable alternative if an oral contraceptive is not recommended. It may be indicated for the woman who finds it difficult to take medications regularly. Prophylactic antibiotics may be necessary when the Norplant is implanted.

- *Intrauterine device* (IUD) can be complicated by local pelvic infections and subsequent generalized infections and is therefore not recommended for any woman at risk for bacterial endocarditis (infections of the heart).

- *Sterilization* (male vasectomy or female tubal ligation) may be recommended when pregnancy is too dangerous for the woman's health.

Family Planning/Genetic Counseling

Both men and women with CHD who are considering starting a family should obtain information about the genetic transmission of CHD well in advance of pregnancy. The risk for genetic transmission overall is very low, but is still higher than in the general population.

The person with CHD and his/her spouse may be referred for genetic counseling for additional guidance and evaluation. An ultrasound or echocardiogram of the fetal heart is recommended usually between the 16th and the 20th week of pregnancy to determine if complex congenital heart disease is present. Ultrasound results can offer reassurance to the parents and/or help determine special needs before or at the time of delivery.

Pregnancy

Many CHD patients tolerate pregnancy well, although pregnancy puts an increased workload on the cardiovascular system. It is very important to discuss this issue with your heart physician *before* becoming pregnant. The potential risks for the woman during pregnancy are determined by the nature of the defect, result of the correction, **and** her overall physical status. Additional heart tests are sometimes needed to evaluate the heart's ability to withstand the extra work of pregnancy. For women planning a pregnancy, certain surgeries may also be done sooner or later than normally planned. In addition, because certain medications can be harmful to the fetus, the physician may need to change some of the medications before conception. Folic acid should be taken daily whenever pregnancy may occur.

Many women with CHD will have a normal pregnancy and delivery. Some women at moderate risk should be followed in a high-risk pregnancy program with her cardiologist, a high-risk obstetrician and an anesthesiologist working together to ensure a safe delivery. Special considerations throughout labor and delivery may be needed, including extra monitoring, additional rest and special medications.

Spontaneous vaginal delivery is usually permitted for women with repaired CHD; Cesarean section is recommended for special obstetrical situations. After delivery, the changes in the woman's body take six to twelve weeks to resolve. The cardiologist may recommend an echocardiogram after this time to assure that the heart has returned to its pre-pregnancy size and function.

For some women with certain congenital heart defects, pregnancy may **not** be advised. This is true for women with a cyanotic defect, pulmonary hypertension, severe heart failure, or fragile blood vessels (e.g., with Marfan's syndrome). In this same group, there may be complications for the fetus also. Babies born to cyanotic mothers are often premature and small for their age.

Menopause

Although many women born with CHD are now in their forties and fifties, there is no specific information available about the effects of congenital heart disease or its treatment on this time in a woman's life. As with the general population, women with CHD should be advised by their physician about hormone replacement therapy.

Family Living

Caring for a child with heart disease, either congenital or acquired, can be both challenging and rewarding. Yet, careful consideration of these tips for family living can greatly reduce the challenges you may face.

Bacterial Endocarditis

Bacterial endocarditis, also known as *SBE (subacute bacterial endocarditis)*, is a serious bacterial infection of the inner lining of heart structures, most often the heart valves. Children and adults with certain congenital or acquired heart defects are sensitive to this infection, although it is extremely rare in people with normal hearts. Symptoms include unexplained persistent low-grade fever, paleness, night sweats, weight loss and a general feeling of illness. When SBE occurs, it often requires a lengthy, expensive, and painful hospital stay, and can make any existing valve damage worse. Thus all efforts should be directed toward prevention.

Anyplace where there is turbulent blood flow, such as a hole in the heart or an abnormal heart valve, bacteria may grow with SBE. The bacteria may settle, multiply, and damage tissue, sending infection into the blood stream (sepsis). Foreign material, such as patches, valves, and tubes, which may be inserted during heart surgery, may also be sources of infection. Dental procedures, especially when oral health is poor (inflamed or infected gums) may also introduce germs into the bloodstream. Children and adults with heart problems should be very careful to maintain good oral hygiene and have frequent dental check-ups.

In order to prevent SBE, the American Heart Association recommends the use of antibiotics prior to any surgery that may cause bleeding. This is especially true of dental, oral, or upper airway procedures, such as removal of tonsils or adenoids, because of their proximity to the heart. With a high level of antibiotic (germ killing medication) in the bloodstream at the time of the procedure, the likelihood of infection is very small. The American Heart Association and the American Dental Association recommend the antibiotic amoxicillin (a prescription medication) by mouth one hour before a dental procedure with no follow-up dose necessary. The administration of antibiotic before a surgical or dental procedure is called SBE prophylaxis.

For procedures within the digestive tract, the esophagus (swallowing tube), and genitourinary tract (bladder, genitals), a combination of intravenous ampicillin and gentamycin is recommended one hour before the procedure begins.

For the normal vaginal delivery of a baby, antibiotics are not recommended.

Some people may be allergic or oversensitive to these drugs, or are supposed to be fasting, or are considered to be a higher than usual risk because of a previous episode of SBE or foreign material in the heart). In that case, other antibiotics may be preferred to be given intravenously. Consult with the cardiologist or dentist to determine the best way to deal with this problem, especially since these recommendations may change from time to time.

At present, loss of loose baby teeth (even with bleeding), skin wounds and other superficial injuries do not require SBE prophylaxis, unless they become badly infected and the physician recommends it. In general, call your cardiologist or cardiac nurse if you are unsure of what to do.

Dental Care Issues

Because of the risk of bacterial endocarditis, children with heart defects need meticulous dental care: cleaning teeth three times a day, flossing, and visiting the dentist regularly. Taking the prescribed regimen of antibiotics prior to any dental procedure is important. Children do not need antibiotic protection when they lose a primary tooth unless there is a special problem.

Like all children, those with heart conditions may need orthodontic treatment. These children's special needs should be discussed with the orthodontist because antibiotic treatment will probably be needed when dental appliances are installed. It is critical to properly clean such appliances to avoid infection over time. Appliances can cause tissue injury during vigorous activities such as contact sports, so these children should wear mouth guards to protect their teeth and prevent damage.

Mouth injuries, abscessed teeth, recurrent canker sores, and accidental tooth loss are all situations that should be discussed immediately with the dentist, who may recommend antibiotics.

A pediatric dentist may be helpful as they often have had direct experience dealing with children who have heart defects and are familiar with the antibiotic regimen. A child who has been through numerous medical procedures may also have some fear of medical personnel. A pediatric dentist may be better able to respond to such a situation.

CPR Training and Renewal

It is recommended that all parents take a course in CPR (cardiopulmonary resuscitation), but it is especially important for parents of a child with heart disease. Follow up with an annual refresher course in CPR is advisable. Many local colleges, park districts, or fire departments offer such classes periodically. Your local hospital or fire department should be able to direct you to programs in your area. The American Heart Association publishes the *Textbook of Pediatric Basic Life Support,* which includes basic instructions on CPR. Written materials, however, should not be used as a replacement for a hands-on course in CPR. They are available to supplement your CPR knowledge.

Fire Department Notification

It is a good idea to notify the local fire department about a child's heart defect if the child is still at all symptomatic or has episodes of arrhythmia, etc. Many parents keep a full description of their child's defect, including a diagram of the child's heart, on file at the local fire department. In this way, paramedics can be alerted to the child's condition as they are en route to the home should there ever be an emergency requiring immediate medical attention.

Preparing for Daycare, School, Camp, etc.

As more children have complete repair of heart defects in infancy or early childhood, fewer of them enter school still needing major cardiac treatment. It is unlikely that any restrictions will be placed on the child's physical activity; most children who have had surgery in infancy can run and play actively. Some children, however, will have some restrictions placed on them by their pediatric cardiologists.

In any event, it is essential for the school to know that surgery has been performed and whether or not full activity is possible. Without specific knowledge, a teacher may be overly anxious and restrict the child's activity needlessly. For children who enter school with a major health problem, their activity will likely be limited, and close coordination between family, school, and cardiologist is critical. When restrictions on physical activity are necessary, alternative ways for the child to participate should be found in order to allow the child to feel as included as possible.

Prior to entering school, there will no doubt be health forms to be completed, and any heart problem or surgery should be described. It is recommended that in addition to this paperwork, a face-to-face meeting with the primary teacher, gym teacher, school nurse, and possibly the principal, be arranged to make sure that they are fully apprised of the child's health and heart history. If the child's physical activity is restricted, ongoing discussions regarding the level of physical activity are most important. It is important for all involved to recognize the subtle differences between challenging, coddling, and embarrassing the child by asking him or her to exceed physical capabilities.

Often the cardiologist will say that a child with a cardiac defect will voluntarily limit himself physically. These children have an exertion point beyond which their bodies will not go; they will be forced to rest. The teacher who is aware of this can make it possible for the child to rest unobtrusively.

Chapter Ten

Preparing for Hospitalization

The hospitalization of a child can be very stressful for everyone involved. Treatment advances now allow many types of illnesses and conditions to be managed on an outpatient basis. But infants and children with congenital heart disease may still require admission to the hospital—to manage new onset congestive heart failure, adjust medication, treat an infection or for diagnostic procedures, just to name a few of many possibilities. Preparing a child, when age-appropriate, and the family will help decrease anxiety and stress for all concerned.

An emergency or unplanned admission, however, leaves little time, if any, for preparation. Families of children with congenital heart disease may want to seek help from their extended families, friends, neighbors, church group or hospital's social services staff during an emergency. Parents and caregivers must focus their attention on the hospitalized child and let others assist with other children, household tasks, etc. It is important to remember that siblings of a hospitalized child are also going through a stressful time and they need their own support systems in place.

Discussing the Hospitalization

The preparation of a child for hospitalization varies depending on the age and cognitive level of the child. Previous hospitalizations also need to be taken into account, and whether they were "good or bad" experiences will be key. No matter what the child's age or previous experience is, however, the parents need to convey a positive attitude when discussing the hospitalization. Statements like, "They'll make you listen in the hospital," or "You'll have to stay in bed all day," should be avoided. Telling children too far in advance about an upcoming hospitalization may cause them to worry unnecessarily. But keep in mind, it is frightening to a child to walk in a room and have the conversation stop or have adults spelling out words.

One rule of thumb for discussing an upcoming hospitalization is to begin explaining what is coming up as many days in advance as the child's age in years. For example, a 2-year-old should be told 2 days ahead of time, and a

5-year-old should be told 5 days in advance. This is a general statement and each family should assess their own child and determine what is best for him or her. Children over the age of 7, in most circumstances, can be told of an upcoming hospitalization as soon as the parents learn about it.

Preparing the Infant

Because an infant cannot understand any explanations of an upcoming hospitalization, preparation is minimal. Separation from parents or caregivers can cause stress and anxiety for a baby. Whenever possible a parent or caregiver should stay with the baby. Bringing a favorite toy, blanket or bottle can help make the infant feel secure and decrease this separation anxiety. Infants can sense parental stress; remaining calm while you are with your child can make the hospital stay easier for everyone.

One way to decrease stress for yourself is to keep well informed about your child's progress. Ask questions and speak with your child's doctors and nurses frequently. In most hospitals, daily "rounds" are made on each patient. While the parents may not be present for the rounds, you can find out afterwards what the plan of care is, the latest test results, and many other aspects of your child's hospitalization that had been discussed. Another way to decrease stress for yourself and your child is to continue to be involved with your child's daily routines while in the hospital. If possible, keep the feeding schedule, nap and play times as close to the home routine as you can. Many times home schedules cannot be followed because of tests, procedures and the like. But sharing your schedule with hospital staff members can be helpful when the plan of care is being discussed. If the staff knows the home routines, they can at least attempt to incorporate them into the hospital stay.

Preparing the Toddler

Toddlers and preschoolers are probably the most difficult group to prepare for a hospitalization. They have a limited comprehension of explanations given to them, and a fear of being separated from their primary caregivers. Toddlers fear the unknown and fear loss of control. Moreover, since that cannot easily verbalize these fears, they often "act out" their fears, by screaming and/or having a tantrum.

To help alleviate these fears, the toddler can be prepared for a hospitalization no more than one to two days ahead of time. Explanations need to be kept very simple and on their level, avoiding words with multiple meanings. Keep the explanations short and, if at all possible, allow your child to touch hospital equipment ahead of time. Many hospital child-life departments have hospital and surgical tours available to you before admission. If these are not available, ask your physician's nurse for a tour.

Whenever possible, minimize the time you will be apart from your child. Bring favorite toys, blankets, etc. to the hospital. This is not the time to buy a new toy and bring it in for the child; he or she needs the comfort and familiarity of things from home. For prolonged stays in the hospital, however, new toys can be brought in to help with the boredom that often sets in.

When a parent does have to leave the hospital, it is helpful to the child if another parent or caregiver remains. When this is not possible, leave something belonging to the parents at the hospital, such as a familiar sweater from mom or dad or a scarf or t-shirt.

It is important to recognize that no matter what preparation was done ahead of time, a hospitalization is going to be stressful. The pediatric staff is familiar with these stressors and often has "tricks of the trade" that they can offer to your family. Do not hesitate to ask for help and accept help from the hospital staff and volunteers.

Preparing the Preschooler

Preschoolers are typically difficult to prepare for a hospitalization. Preschoolers fear bodily injury and mutilation. They are often afraid of the dark and of being left alone. Preschoolers take words very literally and relate them to what they are most familiar with. For example, when explaining surgery, if you use the word "cut," your child may think of taking scissors or a knife and cutting something. Tell him instead that the doctor will fix his heart. If your child has more questions about a hospitalization, ask the hospital staff to help answer them.

Preschoolers generally have vivid imaginations. When you begin preparing your child for hospitalization, usually no more than two to four days prior to the event, you can use your child's imagination to your advantage. Drawing, play-acting or using dolls are some ways to prepare your child. Whatever way you choose, be sure to remain positive and reassure your child that he or she did nothing wrong to cause a problem. Hospitalizations should never be viewed as a form of punishment for the child. Once in the hospital, try to reinforce what was done at home during preparation. Do not assume your child remembers drawing or play-acting. Fear and anxiety often cause the preschooler to forget what was done at home to prepare for coming to the hospital.

Probably one of the most important things to remember when preparing your child for a hospitalization is to tell them the truth. Children remember if they are told, "This will not hurt," or "You won't have to stay overnight." Better to tell your child, "It may hurt, but we'll give you something for the hurt," or "You do have to stay overnight, but I'll stay with you." If you don't tell them the truth, you'll have a difficult time getting your child to trust and believe you the next time.

Don't tie evaluations of your child's behavior to his or her hospitalization. For example, avoid saying, "You're a good boy for holding still." Say instead, "That was good to hold still for the nurse."

After a hospital stay, it is important for children to verbalize or play out their feelings about their stay. Young children often go home and pretend they are still in the hospital. This behavior helps them understand and integrate their hospital experience, as well as help alleviate some of their fears. They are now at home in a safe environment and often feel better about expressing themselves.

Preparing the School Age Child

School age children have some of the same fears as toddlers and preschoolers. In addition, at approximately the age of 7 years, children develop the concept that death is permanent. Their concept of time is emerging, thus leading them to understanding the finality of death. Experiences with death in the family or community or what they see on television help them formulate their concept of death. It is also during this time that they realize their parents are powerless to prevent death. Children at this age often need clarification on the causes of death and reassurance that they are unlikely to die soon.

School age children may be reluctant to ask questions and admit they do not know something. For this reason, they need to have an upcoming hospitalization and procedures explained to them, and then they should be asked to explain what they understand. Children 7 years and older should be told about their hospitalization at least 1 week in advance and allowed to process the information given to them and ask questions. Children at this age learn well with concrete examples and "hands-on" learning. They often like to see and touch equipment that will be used, as well as seeing pictures or using dolls to represent what will happen in the hospital. Many facilities offer hospital tours that allow children to see and touch equipment that will be used, as well as answer questions. Child-life therapists and nurses who deal with children everyday usually conduct these tours and they can be wonderful resources to patients and families.

It is important to remember that a child's cognitive and psychosocial development may not always match his or her chronological age. Development may be delayed in one or both areas. Chronically ill children are particularly at risk, so pre-hospital preparation may need to be adjusted accordingly. Make sure your hospital preparation is done in such a way that your child understands what is being said.

Preparing the Adolescent

Adolescence is a time of change for children. Their bodies are changing and maturing. They are striving for independence and are very involved with their peer group. Adolescents' behavior is often inconsistent and unpredictable. It is normal for them to have mood swings, occasionally be depressed, or exhibit mild antisocial behavior. A hospitalization during this time can be very stressful for everyone involved.

It should never be assumed that an adolescent understands what will happen during a hospitalization, even if he has been hospitalized before. Explanations are very important. Include him in the plan of care. Control is also extremely important to the adolescent, so include him in discussions about a surgery or procedure. Acknowledging your child's frustrations and fears about the hospital stay will help him work through some of his many emotions.

Adolescents are often very self-conscious about their appearance and body image. Assure her that every effort will be made to maintain her privacy while she is in the hospital. She may or may not want to have contact with friends while in the hospital. If she does want friends to visit, give her some visiting time alone with her peers. It will help her to cope better with the hospital stay.

Preparing Yourself

Having a sick child in the hospital is very difficult for families. Whether you have time to prepare for the hospital stay or not, it is important to take care of yourselves during this stressful period. Accept any help that is offered to you and your family. It is important to eat regularly and get rest. Alternate staying at the hospital overnight with other family members, so you can get away from the hospital for a period of time. You need to be ready for your child to come home, when he or she will need you even more. An exhausted, stressed parent will have difficulty being supportive for a hospitalized child.

When you have questions or concerns about your child, don't be afraid to ask. Write down your questions, and even the answers if it helps. Make sure you understand what the various tests and procedures are for and find out about test results. Ask about the medications that are being started or adjusted and what therapies are being administered. You want to be as familiar as possible with your child's care prior to discharge. You are your child's best advocate and you need to stay informed. If you don't understand something, ask to have it explained again until you are comfortable with the answer. If your child has many consulting physicians, ask for a patient care conference. This is a group meeting that involves all the physicians caring for your child, along with you, the primary nurse, and often the unit social worker. The child's hospital course and future plan of care is discussed, and usually discharge concerns are addressed at this time. Many families find these meetings very informative and helpful.

Communicating with family and friends during the hospitalization can be a challenge. Assigning a family member as the go-to person can decrease the amount of phone calls and interruptions. Creating a care page on the hospital's website or via another web base can provide a great way to update multiple friends and family at one time and allow for accurate communications. Reading well wishes can ease the feelings of isolation during a prolonged hospitalization.

When age appropriate, include your child in discussions with his nurses, therapists, physician, and residents, so he can actively participate in his care and understand what is happening. Encourage your child to ask questions and become familiar with his treatments, medications, therapies, the disease process, and surgery. This knowledge will help give him a feeling of control. Let your child be his own advocate, with your support, of course. This can be excellent practice for his future encounters within the health care system.

Although this can be very difficult, you need to try to remain positive about your child's hospitalization whenever you are together. Children pick up on fears and anxiety from their parents and family. The greater the parents' anxiety, the greater the likelihood that the child will have difficulty dealing with hospitalization and illness. If you can, remain positive. It will help your child cope with the hospitalization much better. Studies have shown a correlation between parents' anxiety and the child's difficulty in coping with hospitalization and illness.

Of course, it is perfectly normal to feel anxious and scared. But try to deal with your stress away from your child. Look to your family, friends, community, church group or hospital staff to help you work through your anxiety and fears. But don't hide or ignore your own feelings. You need to be healthy and prepared when your child is discharged home after the hospital stay.

Preparing for Discharge After a Medical Admission
The preparation for your child's discharge should begin shortly after admission to the hospital. Except for prolonged hospitalizations, physicians, nurses, and other hospital personnel will begin discussing plans for sending your child home

almost immediately. The reason for admission will dictate the discharge plans.

Nurses and discharge planners are usually very good about teaching parents what will need to be done at home, but it is never too early to start preparing to take your child home. If your child's care will involve treatments to be done at home—such as dressing changes or insertion of a feeding tube—you should have at least two, preferably three, people learn the routines. Parents or caregivers should learn, as well as a back-up person, such as a baby-sitter or another family member. Other family members or support persons to the family are welcome to come to the hospital to learn about home care.

Care for a sick child should be shared whenever possible, so the primary caregiver doesn't get "burned out." If the child is old enough and capable of doing some of his own home care, encourage his involvement. Children as young as 5 or 6 years old can definitely participate in their own care. If the child is involved, and given explanations as to why things are necessary, he is much more likely to comply with the treatment plan. Children need to be in control of things that are happening to them; doing for themselves gives them that control.

Your discharge instructions should include signs and symptoms to watch for that may indicate a change in your child's condition. Again, if it is age appropriate for your child to be included in these instructions, include her in the teaching. The best person to tell you how your child is feeling is your child.

Make sure you have all of your questions answered before you leave the hospital. Have a follow-up appointment made with the appropriate physicians or a time frame within which a follow-up visit will occur. After discharge, if you have questions or concerns about your child that are not of an urgent nature, write them down for your next physician visit or phone call. Make sure you have contact numbers to call during the day, at night and on the weekends if questions or concerns arise.

If your question or concern is of a more urgent nature, then write it down and call your physician's office. Writing down questions helps you organize your thoughts and remember what it is you need to ask your child's doctor. Many families use a notebook to record their questions and answers as well as hospital discharge papers and instructions so they have the information readily available when further questions arise. This notebook can act as a valuable resource for your child's health history, and be very helpful on subsequent hospital admissions.

Preparing for Discharge After a Surgical Admission

Preparing for discharge after a surgical admission is slightly different from a medical admission. After surgery, care instructions may include care of the incision, bathing, activity restrictions, signs and symptoms of infection and pain management. Each group of surgeons usually has a set protocol for discharge teaching, and many surgical groups have clinical nurse specialists that work with patients and families to help with discharge teaching.

Include your child in the discussion, if age-appropriate, and make sure she understands what the instructions are. Encourage her to ask questions and clarify anything she or you do not understand. Make a follow-up appointment with your surgeon, or know when the appointment should be, before you go home. Generally, one visit with the surgeon after discharge is necessary. This visit is to make sure there are no problems related to the surgery. The incision and sternum (breast bone) may be checked to make sure they are healing properly, the activity and diet of the child may be assessed, and any of your questions should be answered. Unless a complication or problem is identified during this visit, a return visit to the surgeon is usually not necessary. However, if after this visit, a problem or question does come up at home, do not hesitate to call your surgeon or the surgeon's nurse to get an answer.

Once you have seen the surgeon, it is usually recommended that you follow up with your cardiologist within two to four weeks. These time frames can vary, however, so always check with your physician.

At Home Following a Hospitalization

Once you are finally home from the hospital with your child, you may think, "I'm so glad to be home, so everything can go back to normal." Although this is a nice thought, don't expect everything to return to normal immediately after your arrival. Hospital admissions can and do throw off everyone's schedule. Feeding schedules, naps, etc. are often not followed in the hospital and it may take a few days at home to help everyone get back on track. Gradually attempt to get your child back on his home routines. Don't set your expectations too high; it will only frustrate you and your child. Expect his appetite, sleeping patterns and behavior to be altered. Many times after being in the hospital, children come home and don't want to eat or they still aren't feeling well and have little or no appetite. Usually offering them foods they like to eat in small quantities and more frequently works well. If your child is taking medications at home, check with your physician or pharmacist to see if the medications should be given with or without food, then develop a schedule to accommodate this.

Your child may regress in some of his behaviors once he is back home. Children that are toilet trained, for example, may return to needing diapers, especially if this was a recent accomplishment before being admitted to the hospital. Young children may want to start drinking out of a bottle again, and it is not uncommon for parents to notice their children needing more attention once they get home. These are all fairly typical behaviors of children who were recently discharged from the hospital, and all these behaviors do resolve after several days of being back home. Being warned about these behaviors and knowing that they commonly happen—and that they go away—may make the situation easier to tolerate.

Infants who undergo open-heart surgery are at increased risk for neurodevelopmental delays. Close follow-up and screening is recommended for early detection and intervention. Ask your cardiologist about these evaluations. Single-ventricle patients are at increased risk for rehospitalization between surgical interventions. Home monitoring programs are in place to monitor weight gain and oxygen saturations for early detection of any issues. Frequent clinic visits with echo and ECG monitoring can aid in determining the timing of the next surgery.

Sibling Issues

Siblings of hospitalized children often have difficulties of their own that need to be recognized. They often feel left out or forgotten because of the large amount of time that their parents spend at the hospital or talking about the sick child. Depending on the age of the sibling, he or she may not understand what is going on with their brother or sister. She may even feel responsible for the illness or that fighting or arguing with her sibling somehow caused the problem. Siblings can also begin to demonstrate behavioral changes, especially with sleep and eating patterns or school performance.

Siblings should be included in the hospital preparation of the child. If a hospital tour is offered or books are read to the sick child, the siblings should be included, if age-appropriate. Hiding information or not discussing the progress of the child in the hospital can be very scary and upsetting to the sibling. If the hospitalized child is old enough and agrees to visitation, siblings should be allowed to visit. This will help siblings see that the hospitalized child is all right and alleviate some of their fears. As with anyone visiting a patient in the hospital, siblings should be healthy. If they have a cold, sore throat or any symptoms of being sick themselves, they should stay away from the hospitalized child. If they have recently been exposed to a contagious illness at school or daycare they should not visit. Conversely, if the hospitalized child has a viral or bacterial infection, or any other illness that can be transmitted to the sibling, they should not be together. In these situations, phone calls, sending pictures or drawings back and forth, or any other means of communication is preferred over the visitation. Keeping the whole family involved in the hospitalization helps everyone cope during this very stressful time.

Siblings should be encouraged to express their feelings. They often are scared, worried and jealous of the attention their brother or sister is receiving. Spending time with other family members does help, but depending on the age of the child, this will soon be an inadequate substitute for their parents. Although it is difficult when one child is in the hospital, parents should spend time with siblings, too. Parents often feel they need to be at the hospital at all times, and feel guilty about leaving their sick child. Whenever possible, parents should alternate visitation, so one is at the hospital and one can be with the other children. Spending a couple of hours at home can make a big difference to siblings.

Know What's Best For Your Family

These suggestions are only general recommendations. You should evaluate your own situation and decide what is best for you and your children. If you are unsure of what to do, discuss your concerns with the hospital social worker, child-life therapist or nurses caring for your child. They will help you make an informed decision and will help facilitate the visitation.

Hospitalization of a family member is a very difficult time for any family. Uncertainty about the child's illness and fears about the hospitalization are stressful. Take time for yourself. Accept help that is offered to you. Ask questions as they come up. Ask for clarification on anything you don't understand. Keeping yourself, your child and the rest of your family prepared and informed will make things easier to handle in the long run.

Glossary

Glossary of Caregivers

APN (Advanced Practice Nurse) or NP (Nurse Practitioner): An Advanced Practice Nurse is a registered nurse with an advanced masters degree who has specialized in the care of cardiac patients. APNs work closely with the surgeons and cardiologists in managing your child's care.

Attending Physician: A board-certified physician who has completed a residency and fellowship and is a member of the hospital staff. They are in charge of the care of your child.

Cardiologist: A physician who specializes in cardiac care. They may care for your child in the intensive care unit or on the general floor. They may be involved in the management of your child during their hospitalization as well as before and after any procedures.

Cardiac Intensivist: A physician who is specially trained in critical care medicine and cardiology. They are actively involved in managing your child's care during their stay in the intensive care unit.

Cardiac Surgeon: A surgeon who specializes in the care of pediatric congenital heart disease.

EP Cardiologist: A cardiologist with special training in electrophysiology (heart rhythm issues). If your child has any problems or concerns with their heart rhythm, an EP cardiologist may be involved in the diagnosis and treatment and management of your child. They will also manage devices such as a pacemaker or defibrillator if your child requires any of these devices to help control the rhythm of their heart.

Fellow: A physician who has completed their residency and is completing additional training in a specialty area such as cardiology, intensive care, cardiac surgery, or other specialty areas.

Consulting service: If a medical issue arises during your child's hospital stay that is not cardiac related, another specialty may be asked to come and evaluate your child. Other specialty MDs frequently consulted for children with cardiac diagnosis include but are not limited to: pain team, kidney, endocrine, and infectious disease. They help the cardiac team to make sure your child is getting the best care possible. The specialty MD will see your child and may recommend a treatment plan that includes inpatient care as well as outpatient follow-up with their specialty service.

Therapists

Occupational Therapist: Assists with fine motor skills and positioning.

Physical therapist: Assists with muscle coordination and recovering after a prolonged hospitalization that may leave your child with weak muscles.

Respiratory Therapist: Assists with management and maintenance of the ventilator, respiratory supplies and any respiratory treatments your child may require to help them breathe easier.

Speech Therapist: Assists your infant with coordinating sucking and swallowing for infants who struggle with bottle- and breastfeeding during and after hospitalization.

Glossary of Terms

Aneurysm: A ballooning of the wall of a vein or an artery or the heart itself due to weakening of the wall by disease, traumatic injury or an abnormality present at birth.

Angiocardiography: A diagnostic method involving injection of a dye into the bloodstream. Chest x-rays taken after the injection show the inside dimensions of the heart and great vessels, as outlined by the dye.

Anoxia: Literally, no oxygen. This condition most frequently occurs when the oxygen supply to a part of the body is critically diminished. This may result in the death of the affected tissue.

Antiarrhythmic Drugs: Drugs that are used to treat disorders of the heart rate and rhythm, such as lidocaine, procaine amide, quinidine, digitalis, propranolol, atropine, and isoproterenol.

Anticoagulant: A drug that delays clotting (coagulation) of the blood. When given in cases where a blood vessel has been plugged by a clot, an anticoagulant tends to prevent new clots from forming, or the existing clots from enlarging, but does not dissolve an existing clot. Anticoagulants are also used to prevent clots from forming on artificial material, such as artificial valves.

Aorta: The main artery to the body, originating from the base of the heart, arching up over the heart like a cane handle, and passing down through the chest and abdomen near the spine. The aorta normally receives blood from the left ventricle of the heart and moves it to the many lesser arteries that conduct blood to all parts of the body, except the lungs.

Aortic Stenosis: A narrowing at the valve opening, or just above or below the valve, between the left ventricle of the heart and the large artery called the aorta.

Arrhythmia: Any variation from the normal rhythm of the heartbeat.

Arterial Blood: Blood that picks up oxygen in the lungs and normally passes from the lungs to the left side of the heart via the pulmonary veins. This blood is then pumped by the left side of the heart into the arteries that carry it to all parts of the body.

Artery: Any blood vessel that carries blood away from the heart to the various parts of the body. Arteries usually carry oxygenated blood, except for the pulmonary artery, which carries unoxygenated blood from the heart to the lungs, where it picks up oxygen.

Asymptomatic: Without symptoms. A person is considered asymptomatic when he does not exhibit functional evidence of a disease or condition.

Atresia: The absence of a normal opening.

Atrial Septal Defect: An opening in the wall, or septum, that normally divides the left and right upper heart chambers, called the atria.

Atrial Septum: Sometimes called the interatrial septum, this is the muscular wall that divides the left and right upper chambers of the heart, called the atria.

Atrium: Sometimes referred to as the auricle. The atrium is one of the two upper chambers of the heart. The right atrium receives unoxygenated blood from the body. The left atrium receives oxygenated blood from the lungs.

Bacterial Endocarditis: An inflammation of the inner layer of the heart caused by bacteria, sometimes resulting as a complication of another infectious disease, an operation or injury. The lining of the heart valves is most frequently affected, especially valves with previous damage from rheumatic disease or congenital abnormality.

Balloon Angioplasty: A technique accomplished during cardiac catheterization or surgery using a balloon tipped catheter inserted into a vessel, usually to dilate a narrowing or to open a blockage. This is a fairly new procedure.

Balloon Valvuloplasty: A procedure in which a balloon is inserted into the opening of a narrowed heart valve, then inflated to stretched the valve open. When the procedure is complete, the balloon is removed.

Bicuspid Valve: Any valve with two leaflets. The term may refer to a normal mitral valve or an abnormal aortic or pulmonary valve, which normally has three leaflets.

Blood Pressure: The force that flowing blood exerts against the artery walls. Two blood pressures are usually measured: 1)The upper, or systolic, pressure occurs each time the heart contracts to pump blood into the aorta. This part of the heartbeat is called systole; and, 2)The lower, or diastolic, pressure occurs when the heart relaxes and refills with blood. This part of the heartbeat is called diastole. The blood pressure is expressed by two numbers, with the upper one written over the lower one (systolic/diastolic).

Blue Babies: Babies having a blue color of skin, called cyanosis, caused by insufficient oxygen in the arterial blood. This often indicates a heart defect, but may have other causes, such as premature birth or impaired respiration.

Bradycardia: An abnormally slow heart rate. Generally, anything below 60 beats per minute is considered bradycardia.

Bundle of His: Also called the atrioventricular bundle or A-V bundle. This bundle of microscopic specialized fibers lies between the atria and ventricles and is the only known normal direct connection between the atria and the ventricles, serving to conduct impulses to the ventricular heart muscle. It is named after German anatomist Wilhelm His.

Cardiac: Pertaining to the heart. Sometimes refers to a person who has heart disease.

Cardiac Arrest: The cessation of the heartbeat. As a result, blood pressure drops abruptly and circulation of blood ceases.

Cardiologist: A specialist in the diagnosis and treatment of heart disease.

Cardiology: The study of the heart and its functions in health and disease.

Cardiopulmonary Resuscitation (CPR): An emergency measure used by one or two people to artificially maintain another person's breathing and circulation if these functions suddenly stop. CPR is done by keeping the airway open, performing rescue breathing and external cardiac compression, or heart massage, to keep oxygenated blood circulating through the vital organs of the body.

Cardiovascular: Pertaining to the heart and blood vessels.

Carditis: Inflammation of the heart.

Catheter: A thin, flexible tube that can be guided into body organs. A cardiac catheter is made of woven plastic, or other material to which blood will not adhere, and is inserted into a vein or artery, usually of an arm or a leg, and gently threaded into the heart. Its progress can be watched on a fluoroscope.

Catheterization: In cardiology, the process of introducing a thin, flexible tube, called a catheter, into a vein or artery and guiding it through the heart chambers and surrounding vessels for purposes of examination or treatment.

Cineangiocardiography: A diagnostic method similar to angiocardiography, except that instead of still x-ray pictures, motion pictures of the heart are made by fluoroscope as an injected opaque liquid is carried through the heart and blood vessels.

Clubbed Fingers: Fingers with a short broad tip and overhanging nail, somewhat resembling a drumstick. This condition is sometimes seen in children born with certain kinds of cyanotic heart defects and in adults with heart, lung or gastrointestinal diseases. It may also be hereditary and insignificant.

Coarctation of the Aorta: A congenital narrowing of the aorta, the main artery that conducts blood from the heart to the body.

Congenital Anomaly: An abnormality present at birth.

Congenital Heart Defect: Malformation of the heart or of its major blood vessels present at birth.

Congestive Heart Failure: Heart failure is a condition in which the heart is unable to pump the amount of needed blood to the body. This results from any anatomic or chemical abnormality that leads to congestion in the body and/or lung tissues. Congestive heart failure usually develops gradually over several years, although it can be acute (short and severe). It can be treated by drugs and/or, in some cases, by surgery.

Coronary Arteries: The two arteries that arise from the aorta, then arch down over the top of the heart and branch out to provide blood to the working heart muscle.

Cyanosis: Blueness of skin caused by insufficient oxygen in the blood. When hemoglobin is not carrying oxygen, it is dark burgundy and is called "reduced hemoglobin." The blueness of the skin occurs when critical amounts of reduced hemoglobin are present.

Dextrocardia: Abnormal position of the heart within the chest. The heart normally is in the left chest. When dextrocardia is present, the heart is on the right side. This occurs frequently when a congenital heart defect is present.

Diastolic Blood Pressure: The blood pressure inside the arteries when the heart muscle is relaxed.

Digoxin (Digitalis): A drug that causes the heart muscle to pump more effectively, thereby improving the circulation of the blood, and promoting the normal elimination of excess fluid. This drug is often used to treat heart failure. It is also used for certain arrhythmias.

Diuretic: A medicine that promotes the excretion of urine. These drugs are often used to treat conditions involving excess body fluid, hypertension and congestive heart failure. One important class of diuretics is the thiazides.

Ductus Arteriosus: A connection outside the heart of the fetus between the pulmonary artery and body of the fetus. Normally this connection closes soon after birth. If it does not close, the condition is known as patent or open ductus arteriosus.

Dysrhythmia (Arrhythmia): An abnormal rhythm of the heart.

Echocardiography: A diagnostic method in which pulses of high-frequency sound, called ultrasound, are transmitted into the body and the echoes returning from the heart and other structures are made into an electronic picture. These pictures are then studied for diagnostic purposes.

Echo: A picture of the heart and vessels made by echocardiography.

Edema: Abnormally large amounts of fluid in the tissues of the body.

Eisenmenger's Syndrome: A condition in which a large congenital shunting defect is complicated by a pulmonary hypertension, or high blood pressure in the blood vessels of the lungs. A shunting defect is an abnormal opening between the heart chambers, called a septal defect, or between the great arteries, such as patent ductus arteriosus. Some oxygen-poor blood gets pumped to the body and results in cyanosis of the lips, fingernails, and toenails.

Electrocardiogram: Often referred to as ECG or EKG. A graphic record of the electric currents generated by the heart. The word "electrocardiogram" most often refers to a resting electrocardiogram, that is, the patient is lying at rest while the recording is being made. The recording can also be made during exercise or when the patient is walking about.

Endocardial Cushion Defect: A complex congenital heart malformation involving the septum, or wall, between the upper chambers of the heart, called the atria, and the septum, or wall, between the lower chambers of the heart, called the ventricles. The valves between the upper and lower chambers are also malformed.

Endocarditis: An inflammation of the inner lining of the heart or heart valves.

Enlarged Heart: A state in which the heart is larger than normal, most often related to a birth defect or underlying disease. Rarely may represent a normal variant.

Extra Beats/Skipped Beats: Single or multiple irregular beats, or palpitations, usually felt as a skip or momentary cessation of the heartbeat.

Fluoroscope: An instrument for observing the internal body organs at work. X-rays are passed through the body onto a fluorescent screen, where the shadows of the beating heart and other organs can be seen and studied.

Foramen Ovale: A hole between the left and right upper chambers of the heart that normally closes after birth.

Heart Attack: The death of a portion of heart muscle, which may result in disability or death of the individual, depending on the extent of muscle damage. A heart attack occurs when an obstruction in one of the coronary arteries prevents an adequate oxygen supply to the heart. Symptoms may be none, mild or severe, and may include: chest pain, sometimes radiating to the shoulder, arm, neck or jaw; nausea; cold sweat; and shortness of breath or syncope (fainting).

Heart Block: A condition in which the electrical impulse that travels through the heart's specialized conduction system to trigger the events of the heartbeat is slowed or blocked along its pathway. This can result in a dissociation of the rhythms of the upper and lower heart chambers, and is the major disorder for which artificial pacemakers are used.

Heart Disease: A general term used to mean ailments of the heart or blood vessels related to structure or function. May be present at birth (congenital) or developed after birth (functional).

Heart Failure: See Congestive Heart Failure.

Heart-Lung Machine: A special instrument used to provide circulation to the body during open-heart surgery.

Heparin: A type of anticoagulant that is given by injection.

High Blood Pressure: An unstable or persistent elevation of blood pressure above the normal range.

Holter Monitoring: A process by which the ECG can be tape-recorded for 14 hours. The patient wears a small tape recorder connected to electrocardiographic leads placed on the chest for 24 hours. A written diary is kept during that period to record symptoms.

Hypertension: Commonly called high blood pressure. It is blood pressure above the normal range.

Hypertrophy: Enlargement of a tissue or organ due to increase in the size of its cells. This may result from a demand for increased work.

Hypotension: Blood pressure below the normal range. Most commonly used to describe an acute fall in blood pressure as occurs in shock syncope (fainting). It is often called low blood pressure.

Hypoxia: Less than normal content of oxygen in the organs and tissues of the body. At very high altitudes, healthy people experience hypoxia because of the decreased amount of oxygen in the air.

Isoproterenol: A drug that can be used as a cardiac stimulant to treat an abnormally slow heartbeat and to increase the strength of the heart's pumping.

Lanoxin: See Digoxin.

Mitral Valve: The heart valve between the left atrium and left ventricle. It has two flaps, or cusps.

Mitral Valve Insufficiency: An incomplete closing of the mitral valve, which is situated between the upper and lower chambers on the left side of the heart. The mitral valve normally prevents a backflow, or leak, of blood in the wrong direction. Mitral valve insufficiency is sometimes the result of scar tissue that forms after rheumatic heart disease. It can also be caused by a congenital heart defect.

Mitral Valve Stenosis: A narrowing of the mitral valve situated between the upper and lower chambers on the left side of the heart. Sometimes the result of a congenital heart defect.

Murmur: Noise made by blood flow, which may or may not be abnormal.

Open-Heart Surgery: Surgery performed inside the heart with the aid of a heart-lung machine.

Organic Heart Disease: A structural abnormality of the heart or great vessels.

Pacemaker: A small mass of specialized cells in the right atrium of the heart, which gives rise to the electrical impulses that initiate contractions of the heart. Also called the sinoatrial node, or SA node. Under certain circumstances (normal or abnormal), other cardiac tissues may assume the pacemaker role by initiating electrical impulses to stimulate contraction. The term "artificial pacemaker" is applied to an electrical device, which substitutes for a defective natural pacemaker to control the beating of the heart by a series of rhythmic electrical discharges. If the electrodes that deliver the discharges to the heart are placed on the outside of the chest, it is called an "external pacemaker." If they are placed within the chest wall, it is called an "internal pacemaker."

Palpitations: A single or multiple irregular beat usually felt as a skip or momentary cessation of the heartbeat.

Patent Ductus Arteriosus: A congenital heart defect in which a small duct, or tube, between the artery leaving the left side of the heart, the aorta, and the artery leaving the right side of the heart, the pulmonary artery, which normally closes soon after birth, remains open. As a result of its failure to close, blood from the left side of the heart is also pumped into the pulmonary artery and thereby into the lungs. This defect is sometimes called simply patent, or open, ductus.

Patent Foramen Ovale: An oval hole, called the foramen ovale, between the left and right upper chambers of the heart, which normally closes shortly after birth, remains open.

Pericarditis: Inflammation of the membrane sac, the pericardium, which surrounds the heart.

Pericardium: A closed tissue sac surrounding the heart and vessels close to the heart. The space inside the sac, the pericardial cavity, normally contains a fluid, which provides for smooth movements of the heart as it beats.

Persistent Truncus Arteriosus: A congenital cardiac defect, characterized by a single arterial trunk arising from the heart receiving blood from both pumping chambers, the ventricles, and the pulmonary artery.

Prostaglandins: Hormone-like substances made from fatty acids, which are found throughout the body tissues. They are thought to have important roles in tissue metabolism and blood flow.

Pulmonary: Pertaining to the lungs.

Pulmonary Artery: The large artery that normally conveys unoxygenated blood from the lower right chamber of the heart to the lungs. This is the only artery in the body which normally carries unoxygenated blood; all others carrying oxygenated blood to the body.

Pulmonary Edema: Congestion of lung tissues often resulting from critical, congenital, or acquired heart or lung disease.

Pulmonary Hypertension: High blood pressure, or hypertension, in the blood vessels of the lungs. The most common causes are congenital heart defects.

Pulmonary Valve Stenosis: A congenital heart defect in which there is a narrowing of the pulmonary valve, which is situated between the right lower chamber, or the ventricle, and the pulmonary artery.

Pulmonic (pulmonary) Valve: The heart valve between the right ventricle and pulmonary artery. It has three flaps, or cusps.

Radioisotopic Scanning: A diagnostic technique involving radioactive labeling of tissues and organs by the injection of radioisotopes (minimally radioactive material) into the bloodstream. The emitted radioactivity is detected by a scanner and the resulting record of the scan is used to evaluate structural defects or functions.

Regurgitation: The abnormal backward flowing of blood through a valve of the heart.

Rheumatic Heart Disease: A complication of rheumatic fever in which damage results to all layers of the heart, particularly the valves.

Rubella: Commonly known as German measles.

Septa: The muscular walls dividing the two chambers on the left side of the heart from the two chambers on the right. The atrial septum separates the top chambers and the ventricular septum separates the bottom chambers.

SBE: See Bacterial Endocarditis.

Shock: Collapse of the circulation related to a congenital heart defect or acquired heart disease or loss of blood volume.

Shunt: A passage between two blood vessels or between the two sides of the heart, as in cases where an opening exists in the wall that normally separates them. In surgery, a shunt is the operation of forming a passage between blood vessels to divert blood from one part of the body to another.

Sphygmomanometer: An instrument for measuring blood pressure in the arteries.

Stenosis: A narrowing or stricture of an opening. Mitral stenosis, aortic stenosis, etc., means that the valve indicated has become so narrowed that it does not function normally. Also refers to narrowing of a blood vessel.

Stress Test: A diagnostic method used to determine the body's response to physical stress. Usually involves monitoring an EKG and other physiological parameters, such as breathing rate and blood pressure, while the patient is exercising – jogging on a treadmill, walking up and down a short set of stairs, or pedaling on a stationary bicycle.

Subvalvar: Below a valve.

Symptomatic: A person is considered symptomatic when he exhibits functional evidence of a disease or condition.

Systolic Blood Pressure: Pressure inside the arteries when the heart contracts with each beat.

Tachycardia: Abnormally fast heart rate. What is considered tachycardia varies with age.

Tetralogy of Fallot: A complex congenital heart malformation consisting of: 1) an opening in the wall between the lower heart chambers (ventricular septal defect), 2) a narrowing of the pulmonary valve (stenosis) and the muscular area just beneath it, 3) thickening (hypertrophy) of the right ventricle and 4) abnormal position of the great artery (aorta). These children are cyanotic.

Transplantation, Heart: The replacement of a healthy heart from a recently deceased donor into the chest of a person whose own heart can no longer function adequately. The donor's heart then replaces or assists the failing heart.

Transposition of the Great Vessels: A congenital heart defect in which the aorta arises from the right, rather than left, ventricle and the pulmonary artery arises from the left, rather than the right, ventricle. Thus the right heart pumps unoxygenated blood from the body through the aorta and back to the body, and the left heart pumps oxygenated blood from the lungs back to the lungs. Only if there is a sizeable hole between right and left chambers, called a septal defect, or a channel between the aorta and pulmonary artery, patent ductus arteriosus, will enough oxygenated blood get pumped to the body to sustain life. Babies with this condition are critically ill and cyanotic and require surgical correction in the first years of life.

Tricuspid Atresia: A severe congenital heart defect in which the valve between the upper right chamber, the atrium, and the lower right chamber, the ventricle, failed to form. Other associated defects are required for life to persist. These children are cyanotic.

Tricuspid Valve: The heart valve between the right atrium and right ventricle, comprised of three flaps or cusps.

Ultrasound: High frequency sound vibrations, not audible to the human ear. In a sonar-like application, ultrasound can be used by a cardiologist as a diagnostic tool, usually echocardiography.

Valve: An opening covered by membranous flaps between two chambers of the heart or between a chamber of the heart and a blood vessel. When it is closed, blood normally does not pass through.

Valve Conduit: An artificial tubing with an artificial valve used in some congenital heart surgeries.

Valvular Insufficiency: Valves that close improperly and permit a backflow of blood. Valvular insufficiency may result from either congenital or acquired heart disease.

Vascular: Pertaining to the blood vessels.

Vectorcardiography: A special type of EKG.

Vein: Any one of a series of vessels of the vascular system, which carries blood from various parts of the body back to the heart.

Venous Blood: Refers to blood returning to the heart. It is unoxygenated when returning from the body and oxygenated when returning from the lungs.

Ventricle: One of the two main pumping chambers of the heart. The left ventricle pumps oxygenated blood through the arteries to the body. The right ventricle pumps unoxygenated blood through the pulmonary artery to the lungs. Capacity of each ventricle in an adult averages 85 cc or about 3 ounces.

Ventricular Septal Defect: A congenital cardiac defect in which there is an abnormal opening in the wall, or septum, that divides the right and left lower heart chambers, called the ventricles.

Additional Resources

The Children's Heart Foundation
www.childrensheartfoundation.org

American Academy of Pediatrics
www.aap.org

American College of Cardiology
www.cardiosource.org/aac

American Heart Association
www.heart.org

National Institutes of Health
www.nih.gov

National Heart, Lung and Blood Institute
www.nhlbi.nih.gov

Centers for Disease Control and Prevention
www.cdc.gov

Mended Little Hearts
www.mendedlittlehearts.org

Adult Congenital Heart Association
www.achaheart.org

Congenital Heart Information Network
www.tchin.org

Saving Little Hearts
www.savinglittlehearts.com

Kids With Heart
www.kidswithheart.org

Pediheart
www.pediheart.net

Children's Cardiomyopathy Foundation
www.childrenscardiomyopathy.org

Little Hearts
www.littlehearts.org

It's My Heart
www.itsmyheart.org

Hilton Publishing Company
www.hiltonpub.com

Organ Transplant Organizations

Children's Organ Transplant Association (COTA)

  1-800-366-2682

  www.cota.org

National Foundation For Transplants

  www.transplants.org

Organ Donation

  www.organdonor.gov

* please note that Internet site addresses may change without notice